FOCUS ON THE FAMILY RESOURCES

5 KEYS TO SENSIBLE WEIGHT LOSS

PAUL C. REISSER, M.D.

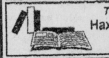

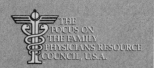

THE FOCUS ON THE FAMILY PHYSICIANS RESOURCE COUNCIL, U.S.A.

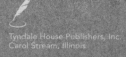

Tyndale House Publishers, Inc.
Carol Stream, Illinois

Visit Tyndale's exciting Web site at www.tyndale.com

TYNDALE is a registered trademark of Tyndale House Publishers, Inc.

Tyndale's quill logo is a trademark of Tyndale House Publishers, Inc.

Living Books is a registered trademark of Tyndale House Publishers, Inc.

Focus on the Family is a registered trademark of Focus on the Family, Colorado Springs, Colorado.

5 Keys to Sensible Weight Loss

Designed by Luke Daab

Adapted from the Complete Guide to Family Health, Nutrition, and Fitness, ISBN-10: 0-8423-6181-2; ISBN-13: 978-0-8423-6181-1. Copyright © 2006 by Tyndale House Publishers, Inc.

ISBN-13: 978-1-4143-1046-6
ISBN-10: 1-4143-1046-3

Printed in the United States of America

12   11   10   09   08   07   06
 7   6   5   4   3   2   1

TABLE OF CONTENTS

FOREWORD BY
DR. JAMES DOBSON

August 15, 1990, began much like any other day for me. I awoke early in the morning and headed to the gym for a game of basketball with a group of friends and colleagues—some of whom were as much as twenty or thirty years younger than I! Because I frequently hit the court with these "youngsters," and because I had reached middle age with the lanky build that allowed me to still move easily, I assumed that I was in the prime of physical health.

A sharp pain in my chest on that late summer morning told me otherwise. I excused myself from the game and drove alone to the hospital (something I do *not* recommend to anyone who suspects he or she is experiencing a serious medical problem!). Hoping and praying that I was merely battling fatigue, I knew deep down that there was something else terribly wrong. It didn't take the doctors long to confirm that, sure enough, this "healthy" basketball enthusiast had transformed, in the blink of an eye, into a heart attack victim.

As I lay in the hospital in the days following that ordeal, I realized that, early-morning basketball games notwithstanding, my predicament was directly related to my lifestyle choices and, in particular, the fatty foods I was allowing in my diet. I asked the Lord to give me another chance, resolving to use every resource at my disposal to safeguard my heart and my health through a combination of healthy diet and exercise. Despite some setbacks (I suffered a stroke in 1998 but recovered from it almost immediately), I have endeavored to keep that commitment, and, today, I am feeling better than ever.

Like so many Americans, prior to my heart attack, I was extremely busy—but not necessarily *active* in a way that would ensure optimal physical health. Indeed, statistics show that, despite our frantic pace of living and continued advances in the medical field, Americans suffer from an alarming number of health problems, many of which could be prevented or at least decreased by changing bad habits.

Research confirms just how serious the situation has become. The latest figures from the American Heart Association show that 13 million Americans have coronary heart disease; 5.4 million have suffered a stroke; and 65 million have been diagnosed with high blood pressure. Unfortunately, a large number of these cases are related, at least in part, to lifestyle choices. The AHA also reports that 48.5 million American adults (nearly 23 percent) are smokers. From 1995 to 1999, an average of 442,398 Americans died annually of smoking-related illnesses (32.2 percent of these deaths were cardiovascular related). The American Cancer

Society estimates that 180,000 of the cancer deaths in 2004 could be attributed to smoking. Further, one-third of cancer deaths in 2004 were related to nutrition, physical inactivity, being overweight or obese, and other lifestyle issues. In other words, many of them were *preventable*!

As I suggested earlier, perhaps the biggest factors in maintaining proper physical health are diet and exercise. Unfortunately, a recent study revealed that a full 25 percent of Americans reported participating in *no* physical activity during their leisure time. Perhaps that is why more than 65 percent of adults in the United States are overweight, including 30 percent who are clinically obese. Between 1971 and 2000, the average daily caloric intake for men grew by about 7 percent, which translates into seventeen pounds of additional body fat per year. Obesity dramatically affects life span, as well. The life expectancy of a twenty-year-old white male who is clinically obese decreases by an estimated thirteen years, and for black males, an astonishing average of twenty years are lost due to obesity. One recent study revealed that the number of annual deaths attributable to obesity among adults in the United States is about 300,000. And perhaps most telling of all, airlines are telling us that they now have to carry additional fuel in order to transport more overweight customers.

This situation is sobering, but I am living proof that a dramatic change in eating habits, combined with a focused regimen of heart-strengthening exercise, can significantly improve one's overall health. I'll admit that the prospect of making such radical lifestyle changes can be daunting, but let me assure you that it is worth the investment. Choosing a healthy lifestyle *now*, while you still can, is infinitely preferable to being sidelined by a stroke, heart attack, cancer, or some other health crisis in the future.

This pocket guide and its parent book, the *Complete Guide to Family Health, Nutrition, and Fitness*, are excellent resources designed to answer many of the questions that may arise as you endeavor to put yourself and your loved ones on the road to a healthier life. You'll find information on preventing the three most common health problems—cardiovascular disease, cancer, and diabetes—as well as practical advice on those critical disciplines that I have mentioned several times already: *diet and exercise*. These books can help you discover answers to specific health-related questions for family members of all ages; foster *emotional* and *spiritual* health in addition to physical fitness; and so much more. The information presented here is based on the most up-to-date medical research as well as the firsthand experiences of members of Focus on the Family's Physicians Resource Council.

Perhaps you consider yourself generally healthy and are simply looking for a plan to help you stay that way. Or maybe you or someone you love is dangerously overweight or suffering from a serious health problem related to poor lifestyle choices in the past. Either way, this book will provide you with the tools you need—as a complement to the advice of your personal physician, of course—to live smarter and healthier. Change is never easy, but it *is* possible, and I pray that God will bless you as you endeavor to be a good steward of the body He has given you.

James C. Dobson

James C. Dobson, Ph.D.

ACKNOWLEDGMENTS

The following members of the Focus on the Family Physicians Resource Council served as primary reviewers for all or parts of this manuscript, and their input, suggestions, and insights have been of critical importance:

BYRON CALHOUN, M.D., F.A.C.O.G., F.A.C.S.
Maternal-Fetal Medicine—Rockford, Illinois

DOUGLAS O. W. EATON, M.D.
Internal Medicine—Loma Linda, California

ELAINE ENG, M.D., F.A.P.A.
Psychiatry—Flushing, New York

J. THOMAS FITCH, M.D., F.A.A.P.
Pediatrics—San Antonio, Texas

DONALD GRABER, M.D.
Psychiatry—Elkhart, Indiana

W. DAVID HAGER, M.D., F.A.C.O.G.
Gynecology—Lexington, Kentucky

DANIEL R. HINTHORN, M.D., F.A.C.P.
Infectious Disease—Kansas City, Kansas

GERARD R. HOUGH, M.D., F.A.A.P.
Pediatrics—Brandon, Florida

GAYLEN M. KELTON, M.D., F.A.A.F.P.
Family Medicine—Indianapolis, Indiana

JOHN P. LIVONI, M.D.
Radiology—Little Rock, Arkansas

ROBERT W. MANN, M.D., F.A.A.P.
Pediatrics—Mansfield, Texas

MARILYN A. MAXWELL, M.D., F.A.A.P.
Internal Medicine/Pediatrics—St. Louis, Missouri

PAUL MEIER, M.D.
Psychiatry—Richardson, Texas

GARY MORSCH, M.D., F.A.A.F.P.
Family Medicine—Olathe, Kansas

MARY ANNE NELSON, M.D.
Family Medicine—Cedar Rapids, Iowa

GREGORY RUTECKI, M.D.
Internal Medicine—Columbus, Ohio

ROY C. STRINGFELLOW, M.D., F.A.C.O.G.
Gynecology—Colorado Springs, Colorado

MARGARET COTTLE, M.D.
Palliative Care—Vancouver, British Columbia

PETER NIEMAN, M.D., F.A.A.P.
Pediatrics—Calgary, Alberta

TYNDALE PUBLISHER

DOUGLAS R. KNOX

ACKNOWLEDGMENTS

EDITORIAL STAFF

PAUL C. REISSER, M.D.
Primary Author

DAVID DAVIS
Managing Editor/Contributing Author

LISA JACKSON
Tyndale Editor

FOCUS ON THE FAMILY

BRADLEY G. BECK, M.D.
Medical Issues Advisor/Research Editor/Contributing Author

VICKI DIHLE, PA-C
Medical Research Analyst/Contributing Author

BARBARA SIEBERT
Manager, Medical Outreach

LINDA BECK
Administrative Support

REGINALD FINGER, M.D.
Medical Issues Analyst

KARA ANGELBECK
Health and Wellness Coordinator

TOM NEVEN
Book Editor

IF YOU WANT TO LOSE WEIGHT

I hate what I see in the mirror.

I can't fit into any clothes.

Normal-sized seats on an airplane or at a theater are uncomfortable or just too small for me.

My love life is nonexistent.

People don't treat me with respect, or if they do, they're just acting.

I've done every diet program on the planet, and I always gain back whatever I lose, with some extra pounds for good measure.

I'm such an utter failure.

For every person whose life is seriously affected by weight (and whose prevailing thoughts and feelings are as dark as these), there are many more who are annoyed and frustrated by a dozen or two extra pounds that they can't ever seem to shed. There are also a significant number who are overweight but not particularly concerned about it—at least until the doctor, or an episode of chest pain, sounds the alarm.

Speaking of alarms, the impact of excessive weight extends far beyond personal image or social acceptance, as important as those issues are. According to the American Obesity Association, it has been estimated that, as a nation, the United States is more than 2.5 billion pounds overweight. The health fallout is staggering: Overweight and obesity may soon overtake smoking as the leading cause of excess death in this country. America's mushrooming weight problem has morphed from a nagging concern into a four-alarm fire among health professionals and federal policy makers alike. This is all well and good, and we will no doubt benefit in a number of ways from attending to this problem as a nation. But for now many of us have some important work to do as individuals.

Whether you are squaring off against a weight problem for the first time, or feel like an old pro with a line of notches in your belt for all of the programs that you've tried without success, what you'll find in this book is some hope: No matter what your scale says, no matter how long you've struggled, no matter how many times you've lost weight only to see it come back again (or even rise higher than ever), it's *never* too late to make changes that will have an impact on your weight, your health, and your sense of well-being. If you don't have a weight problem yourself, you no doubt know many others who do—including, perhaps, your spouse or one or more of your children. This book will offer some ideas that can help you give them both encouragement and practical support—along with a little basic training and a fair number of reality checks. The latter aren't terribly common in many best-selling, surefire, fat-melting miracle diet books, programs, and supplements that swallow billions of our hard-earned dollars every year. If any of these are actually working for you, by all means stay with them. For the other 95 percent of you, read on.

1

AM I OVERWEIGHT
OR OBESE?

You might think that your mirror answers this question, but in fact the boundaries between normal and excessive weight have long been a thorny issue for nutrition experts and the general public alike. In order to get the most out of this book, you should know something about some widely used (and also useful) definitions of *overweight* and *obese*.

BODY FAT PERCENTAGE

We need to remember that our concern about weight is rarely focused on the bone, muscle, internal organs, and other miscellaneous tissue that are all part of our weight, but rather on excess fat.

How much fat is too much? One basic approach to this question is to consider your body fat percentage. How much of your total body weight consists of fat tissue? As a rule of thumb, a healthy adult male carries 12 to 20 percent body fat, and a healthy female 20 to 30 percent. (The difference between genders is a by-product of changes during sexual maturation, as women acquire fat in breasts and hips under the influence of estrogen, while men more readily gain muscle mass in response to testosterone.) For a highly conditioned athlete, these numbers may be cut in half. At the other end of the spectrum, health problems are associated with:

- More than 22 percent body fat in younger men.
- More than 25 percent in men over forty.
- More than 32 percent in younger women.
- More than 35 percent in women over forty.

A time-honored, low-tech method of estimating body fat involves taking skinfold measurements. A fold of skin in any of several locations—most commonly the triceps, or underside of the upper arm—is pulled away from underlying muscle, and its width is measured using a calibrated device called calipers. The measurements are plugged into a formula to obtain the body fat estimate. The accuracy of this approach may be compromised by variations in technique, quality of calipers used, extremes in body fat, and even the basic assumption that fat under the skin in various locations accurately reflects total body fat.

There are a number of more sophisticated technical approaches to measuring body fat percentage, but many of these tests are expensive to perform and not available to the average individual. However, one measurement that estimates the percentage of body fat, known as bioelectrical impedance, can be done using devices available in some health clubs and doctors' offices, although it is less accurate in severely obese individuals. These instruments measure the resistance to the flow of a harmless (and painless) electrical signal between two points in the body. Based on the fact that current flows more readily through some tissues than others (fat in particular does not conduct well), the devices calculate an estimate of body fat percentage. (Note: Bioelectrical impedance varies with a person's level of hydration and will overestimate body fat content if a person is dehydrated. When tracking progress over time, the most reliable results are obtained if measurements are carried out under similar conditions—at roughly the same time of day, for example, and with proper hydration.)

Knowing your body fat percentage can be motivating (especially if you have a lot of weight to lose), but it isn't that useful for week-to-week monitoring. For that job we rely on the scale. Not surprisingly, there has been considerable research on the relationship between height, weight, body fat, and health.

BODY MASS INDEX (BMI)

In recent years, the body mass index, or BMI, has become a widely used tool for determining a healthy body weight. Your BMI, which is based on your current height and weight, is calculated using the following formula:

$$BMI = \frac{weight\ in\ kilograms}{(height\ in\ meters)^2}$$

Since few people in the United States know their weight in kilograms or height in meters, the formula can be adapted for the more familiar pounds and inches system used in the United States:

$$BMI = \frac{weight\ in\ pounds}{(height\ in\ inches)^2} \times 703$$

Those who don't want to do the math can find BMI calculators on several Web sites. Two of these are http://nhlbisupport.com/bmi/bmicalc.htm (courtesy of the National Heart, Lung, and Blood Institute) and http://www.cdc.gov/nccdphp/dnpa/bmi/calc-bmi.htm (Centers for Disease Control and Prevention, or CDC). Type in your height and weight, hit the button that says "calculate" or "compute," and you'll get the answer.

So what does the body mass index tell us? It correlates with body fat—not perfectly, but well enough to serve as a general indicator of the health risk associated with our weight. In 1998 the National Institutes of Health established the following categories for weight based on BMI among adults twenty years and older. These are now widely utilized among health professionals and researchers:

BMI	Weight Status
Below 18.5	Underweight
18.5 to 24.9	Normal
25.0 to 29.9	Overweight
30.0 to 39.9	Obese
Over 40.0	Extremely obese

The BMI is an important and useful number—and you should know yours—but there are some important things to keep in mind. The BMI calculation for an adult is based solely on height and weight, without reference to age or sex. This makes it easier to use—no need for separate calculations and tables for men and women, for example—but the relationship between BMI and "fatness" is not absolute. Women tend to have a higher percent of body fat than men with the same BMI, and older adults are likely to have more body fat than their younger counterparts with the same BMI. A young male bodybuilder might have a BMI of 27, which is classed as overweight, but he may actually have a lot of lean body mass (i.e., bulging muscles), so he would not be considered to have an excess of body fat.

Keep in mind that the various categories of BMI—normal, overweight, and so on—are not absolute boundaries. Experts have argued back and forth about where to draw these lines, and there is not a sudden transformation in health status when a few pounds of weight loss bring a person from a BMI of 30 to 29.9, or from 25 to 24.9. Health risks generally rise with increasing BMI, and do so more dramatically as the BMI climbs past 30. In medical literature, a person with a BMI of 40 or more is said to have *morbid obesity*, reflecting the significant number of health problems associated with this level of excessive weight.

Also note that these categories do not apply to children and teenagers. Between the ages of two and twenty, excessive weight is based not only on BMI but also on age and gender. Your child's physician or dietitian can determine whether he or she has a weight problem using height and weight measurements along with standarized *BMI-for-age growth charts*.

APPLES AND PEARS

Weight-loss experts characterize overweight people as apple- or pear-shaped based on their fat distribution. Those with a prominent abdomen—shaped somewhat like apples—are thought to be at higher risk for health problems than those shaped like pears, with more fat deposited in the hips and thighs.

Two simple measurements related to apple and pear shapes tell us something about a person's health risk:

- **The waist circumference,** measured as the distance around the smallest area above the umbilicus (belly button) and below the rib cage. A measurement of more than forty inches in men and thirty-five inches in women is a cause for concern, because it suggests the presence of excessive fat within and around the abdomen. Fat stored here (a pattern more common in men) should be considered more dangerous to health than fat stored in the hips and thighs (a pattern more common in women). Note that waist circumference is a less meaningful measurement in adults five feet or under or with a BMI of 35 or more.

- **Waist-to-hip ratio** is another way to look at health risk from fat by comparing the amount of fat stored in the abdomen with the amount gravitating toward the hips and thighs. The waist circumference is measured as above, while the hip circumference is measured around the widest portion of the buttocks. Dividing waist by hip circumference gives the ratio, which ideally should be 0.90 or less in men and 0.80 or less in women. As you might expect from knowing that abdominal fat is more troublesome, a ratio of 1.0 or more (reflecting an apple- rather than a pear-shaped individual) suggests a greater health risk.

Several studies have suggested that an increased waist-to-hip ratio is associated with an increased risk for diabetes, high blood pressure, and coronary artery disease. However, compared to the waist-to-hip ratio, the waist circumference appears to be both a better indicator of abdominal fat content and a better predic- tor of future health problems. Indeed, waist circumfer- ence gives you an independent picture of your health risk above and beyond that of your BMI. For example, you should be concerned if your waist circumference is in the higher risk range (over forty inches for men, over thirty-five inches for women), even if your BMI is in the normal or modestly overweight range. However, if your BMI is over 35, measuring waist circumference offers little benefit, other than helping you decide what clothes are likely to fit.[1]

[1]National Institutes of Health, *Clincial Guidelines on the Identification, Evalua-tion, and Treatment of Overweight and Obesity in Adults—The Evidence Report,* NIH Publication No. 98-4083 (September 1998): 56–8.

2

IS IT WORTH THE EFFORT TO LOSE WEIGHT?

Before embarking on a weight-loss plan, it's important to identify your reasons for losing weight. We say *your* reasons because too many people try to lose weight in order to please someone else or to get another person (especially a spouse, a relative, or even a physician) off their back. This may provide motivation for a while, but it rarely sustains a long-term effort because resentment and resistance nearly always enter the picture. Sooner or later you need to identify, write down, and repeatedly review what it is about losing the weight that will keep you going when the going gets tough.

Big important hint to spouses and parents: If you don't like your wife's, husband's, or child's current weight, the best way to make matters *worse* is to provide a steady stream of criticism and sarcastic comments about his or her appearance. Believe it or not, he or she is well aware of this problem, and the last thing needed is another critic to chime in with the one already sounding off day and night in his or her mind. If you want to help, you need to become that person's most steadfast source of love, support, reassurance, and safety. From that position you may then exercise the option (or in the case of a minor child, the responsibility) to express your heartfelt concern and your willingness to help in any way possible. Your message cannot be, *I can't love you at this weight,* but rather, *I love you too much to see you hurt—or your life threatened—by this problem.*

ADJUST, AMEND, OR ELIMINATE ANY COUNTERPRODUCTIVE EXPECTATIONS AND BELIEFS

This is the most important part of the process. Here are some key things to keep in mind—and keep on keeping in mind:

Learn to appreciate slow and steady progress. Fad diets and supplements always promise rapid and spectacular weight loss, and many career dieters cycle in and out of programs in a futile effort to lose twenty pounds by summer or to fit into a special outfit for a big occasion. Repeated cycles of weight loss and gain, often called yo-yo dieting, may actually cause your body to become more resistant to losing weight the next time you try. *Reality check:* The most reliable weight loss occurs *gradually*. A pound or two every week is very good progress. More than two pounds a week on an ongoing basis is uncommon and more likely to be hazardous. Many people lose a few pounds of fluid during the first several days of calorie restriction. But once the water has passed, slower, steady weight loss should be the rule.

Adopt realistic expectations. If you're nearing fifty and want to weigh what you did in college, think again. If you're looking at the models in the department-store ads or the muscular hulks in the typical men's-health magazine and want to be like them, good luck. Beyond whatever physical gifts God provided them, most of them spend a lot of time developing that look (and get a bit of help from photo enhancement techniques), which is likely to be beyond the reach of most mortals. *Reality check:* Your primary goal should be to arrive at a weight that improves your health and sense of overall well-being. For most adults the primary target will be a weight that gives you a BMI of 25. You can check one of the BMI calculators mentioned on page 4 as a point of reference, but you should also determine with your doctor or a registered dietitian whether that weight is in fact optimal for you. Remember also that if you are significantly overweight (that is, a BMI over 30), even a modest loss of 5 or 10 percent can make a major difference in some important risk factors, including cholesterol, triglycerides, blood sugar, and blood pressure.

Embrace your life in the present. If you are perpetually discontented and think that losing weight will change everything, think again. Yes, there are personal and social benefits associated with being at a healthy weight, but if you're never satisfied with your life at your current weight, it's unlikely that your life minus several pounds will be much better. There are plenty of beautiful, thin, miserable people who can attest to this fact. *Reality check:* True happiness is an "inside job," one that unfortunately eludes too many who seek it in all the wrong places. Remember, for starters, that God loves you unconditionally in the body you inhabit *now*.

Take personal responsibility. If you continually blame your genes, your parents, fast-food restaurants, the sugar industry, or anyone else for your weight problem, you're wasting some perfectly good energy. *Reality check:* The bad news is that no one can lose weight for you. The good news is that no one can stop you from losing weight.

Realize that losing weight is not a prison sentence. We often approach the day before we launch another weight-loss plan with dread and a self-defeating last grasp at food freedom: "Eat, drink, and be merry, for tomorrow we die(t)." Some consume impressive amounts of their favorite guilty pleasures, assuming that the next stretch of life is going to be a dry, dusty trail of deprivation. Indeed, the phrase "I'm going on a diet" carries a lot of emotional baggage: "I'm going to serve a sentence for my wrongdoing. When I'm done being punished, though, I'll be free again to do what I like." *Reality check:* Weight management requires an established pattern you can live with for the rest of your life. For some, this may feel like facing life in prison, but such a perspective needs to be tossed aside immediately, because only the most iron-willed individual can adhere to a program that involves perpetual hunger or a list of foods that make you gag. Believe it or not, a healthy diet can be one that allows you to lose weight, nourish your body, avoid hunger, and provide some eating pleasure as well. What you may not be able to find, however, is an approach that does all of these while soothing every emotional discomfort in your life. One of the biggest accomplishments of squaring off against excessive weight is figuring out ways to manage the stresses of life without reaching for food. More on that topic later.

Learn and grow from your mistakes. Nearly everyone with long-term weight problems has felt as if an endless refrain of the pop song "Oops! . . . I Did It Again" is playing. Whether you're attempting a well-reasoned eating plan or the latest fad diet, after a few days or weeks there's an inevitable slip—typically at the end of a hectic, stressed-out, exhausting day. The old comfort food beckons and there's no resisting it. The next day brings a barrage of mental accusations: *I blew it so badly last night. I just erased all of my efforts from the last three weeks, so there's no point in continuing this. Reality check:* If you think unbroken perfection is the only path to success with weight loss, take a moment to consider anything else you've ever accomplished or attempted: walking as a toddler (okay, you don't remember, but you've seen the pictures), reading, spelling, throwing a ball, driving a car, becoming a husband or wife, raising a child, gaining spiritual maturity. If you haven't experienced frustration, failures, and setbacks, you haven't accomplished anything. Furthermore, in the realm of weight loss and gain, what happens at one meal or in one day has far less impact on your weight than the ongoing pattern of food choices.

Be encouraged. You can succeed! You may be frustrated, but "I'll never be able to lose weight" is a blues refrain you can't afford to be singing. *Reality check:* No matter how many times your weight seems to have defeated your efforts, you can make changes that will move this problem in the right direction.

3

THE FIRST KEY: STOP LOOKING FOR THE QUICK FIX

Whether your weight is a relatively new problem or you've tried everything without any long-term success, it's never too late to do something about it. If you're determined to do something about your weight, good for you! But you have an important decision to make at the outset, *especially* if you have struggled with weight for years and already feel utterly frustrated. Whatever else you do, get rid of the expectation that there is some supplement, medication, combination of foods, machine, or fifteen-minute exercise that will magically solve this problem for you. The fact that there are so many different books, programs, and supplements all claiming to have the answer, and at the same time there are so many overweight people desperately looking for something that *really works,* tells you that (at least for now) there is no universal quick and easy cure for this problem.

Navigating the myriad weight-loss programs available

can be quite difficult. But armed with some perspective on current trends in weight loss and a healthy dose of skepticism, you can decide whether the latest diet best seller or surefire diet plan beckoning from the magazine at the supermarket checkout line is potentially worthwhile or a lot of hype.

FAD DIETS

Fad diets are a diverse group of eating or weight-loss plans with one or more of the following characteristics:

- **A premise that doesn't make scientific or nutritional sense.** Example: Books that claim the right diet for you depends on your blood type, an idea so eccentric that no reputable scientific organization (or even the vast majority of alternative practitioners) takes it seriously.
- **Claims that the diet is "unique," "groundbreaking," "a breakthrough," etc.** Translation: "I thought this up myself."
- **Extreme restrictions or a focus on a single "miracle" food that boosts metabolism, burns fat, etc.** Examples: the grapefruit diet, the cabbage soup diet, the peanut butter diet, the chicken soup diet, and the apple cider vinegar diet. (There's even a chocolate diet!) Any of these may work for a while, based on two principles. First, if you can eat only one or a handful of foods, after a while you don't look forward to eating, except as a way to curb hunger. (Before long, of course, you'll get sick of the whole thing and toss the diet overboard.) Second, some of these diets tell you to eat smaller portions, exercise more, avoid sugary and rich foods, and (by the way) be

sure to eat the featured food every day. Guess which component of the diet actually results in weight loss?

- **Diets invented or endorsed by a celebrity.** They may be sensible or silly, but they depend on a basic craving of many overweight people: "If only I could look just like _____."

- **Diets that involve "food-combining" or other convoluted restrictions.** Example: Diets that claim you shouldn't eat fruits with other types of food, or that you shouldn't combine starches and vegetables at the same meal, or that you *can* combine starches and vegetables as long you don't add fat, and so on. Usually these diets are based on the ideas of some obscure author of a century or so ago, and none are consistent with solid nutritional science. They also tend to imply that following their particular formula is the best (or only) way for us to enjoy good health. Here's a question to ask of all food-combining diets: *How in the world did the human race survive (let alone lose weight) before this diet was published?*

- **Diets that claim to "detox" (detoxify) your body.** The prospect of detoxifying the body has a lot of appeal both for people trying to lose weight and for those suffering from fatigue or other chronic complaints. The premise goes something like this: Chemicals that pollute our air, water, seas, and soil have found their way into our food (or they have been put there during modern processing) and have accumulated in our body. Our ability to eliminate them is hampered by poor food quality, stress, and a number of other factors, resulting in weight gain, fatigue, depression, headaches, bowel problems, arthritis, and even cancer. We may be harboring harmful organisms such as *Candida albicans*, which release more toxins into the body. This state of toxicity is said to be treatable using a stringent combination of raw fruits and vegetables, a water or juice fast, supplements, herbs, colon cleansing (including enemas), and perhaps other treatments as well, including massage, breathing exercises, aromatherapy, and so on. Words such as *flushing, cleansing, neutralizing, elimination,* and even *scrubbing* (as in, "our product will scrub out your cells") are used frequently, bringing to mind a spring cleaning of the body, after which health and well-being (not to mention weight loss) will follow. All sorts of detox programs are marketed on the Internet, in health-food stores and spas, and via infomercials, often with price tags as impressive as their claims.

Alas, while the detox concept provides some appealing mental imagery, otherwise it is at best vague and at worst mythological. The promoters of these diets and programs never identify, let alone measure, the actual toxins that are supposedly being eliminated. None can offer any reasonable biological explanation of how their diet, supplements, or treatments remove toxins or help the body perform this function. There is no coherent body of research that demonstrates or remotely proves the existence of a detox process as described by these individuals and companies. The words may be different, but the twenty-first-century pitch bears a striking resemblance to the nineteenth-century medicine show, and in both cases the marketing horse is many miles out of the scientific barn.

Bottom line: There's nothing wrong with getting back to basics with some wholesome fruits and vegetables, and cutting back on the processed foods and megaportions. You will feel better, but you don't need to buy into (literally) a lot of supplements, enemas, and half-baked theories to get this result.

LOW-FAT/HIGH-CARBOHYDRATE DIETS

A few decades ago researchers concluded that elevated blood cholesterol was associated with an increased risk for diseased arteries, heart attack, and stroke. Furthermore, foods containing fat tend to be more calorie dense—fat, after all, contains nine calories per gram, while carbohydrates and protein contain four calories per gram. Therefore, if you want to lose weight and avoid having a heart attack, avoiding fat would be a good idea, right?

"Reduce your intake of fat" has in fact been advised for decades, but some have promoted this idea as the main event, the first commandment both for health and healthy weight. The most widely quoted proponent of a fat-restricted diet is Dean Ornish, M.D., founder and director of the Preventive Medicine Research Institute in Sausalito, California, and author of several books, including *Eat More, Weigh Less*. He advocates a very low-fat diet (less than 10 percent of total calories from fat) that is plant based—whole grains, fruits, and vegetables—except for nonfat dairy products and egg whites. All meats, oils, and products that contain oils, nuts and seeds, olives, avocados, and any commercial product containing more than 2 grams of fat per serving are to be avoided or eaten as little as possible. While his 1990 book *Dr. Dean Ornish's Program for Reversing Heart Disease* gave a green light to nearly any type of carbohydrate, more recently he has discouraged sugar and refined/processed carbohydrates.

His comprehensive program for patients with coronary disease includes moderate exercise, stress management, and group support. He has published controlled studies in reputable medical journals demonstrating weight loss and even reduction of coronary artery disease among patients who adhere closely to his program. How much of their improvement is specifically related to diet (as opposed to the other elements of his program) is unclear, although Dr. Ornish advocates forcefully for the entire package.

Another low-fat program was popularized by inventor Nathan Pritikin, who in 1956 discovered that his blood cholesterol level was well above 300. He then failed a stress test, suggesting the presence of significant coronary artery disease. Facing this grim situation at the age of forty-one, he questioned the prevailing medical advice of that time, which in essence said, "Don't exercise, don't climb stairs, take naps, and don't bother changing your diet because you can't control your own cholesterol." Instead, he embarked on a vegetarian diet and a rigorous program of walking and jogging. By 1960 his cholesterol was a mere 120 and a follow-up stress test was normal.

Encouraged by these results, Pritikin initiated a number of research projects, wrote several books (including *The Pritikin Program for Diet and Exercise*), and in 1975 opened the Pritikin Longevity Center. Now located in Aventura, Florida, the Center has hosted some 75,000 guests, who spend one or two weeks in a resort-like setting to initiate lifestyle changes based on Pritikin's dietary and exercise principles. The diet is similar to that advocated by Dr. Ornish, though a single small serving of lean meat is allowed every day. Dozens of research studies in mainstream scientific journals have documented a number of medical benefits, including weight loss, reduced cholesterol and triglycerides, and improved control of diabetes among individuals who have followed this or a similar dietary and exercise approach. After Nathan Pritikin's death in 1985, his autopsy reportedly revealed that he was free of coronary artery disease.

Nathan Pritikin's son Robert now carries his father's low-fat torch, but he has reframed it somewhat in what he calls the Calorie Density Solution. In the book *The Pritikin Principle*, he advocates eating foods that have a low-calorie density—that is, fewer calories per pound—without going hungry or worrying about portions. As you might imagine, fruits, vegetables, beans, and unprocessed grains have much lower calorie densities than highly processed, fatty, and sugary foods. (A pound of broccoli, for example, contains a mere 130 calories, while a pound of chocolate chip cookies packs more than 2,000.) Low-density foods, many of which have a lot of fiber, generally create a sense of fullness (especially if a generous amount of water is part of the meal), and so Pritikin claims that one can eat them freely without worrying about portions or going hungry. The book lists hundreds of foods according to their calorie density, and following the program involves keeping the average calorie density for a meal below a certain level. He also recommends walking thirty miles a week, or more than four miles per day—a worthy goal, but at a brisk pace this represents at least an hour of walking every day.

Advantages: There can be little doubt that someone who perseveres on a diet consisting of vegetables, fruits, unprocessed grains, and very little fat can nearly always expect to lose weight and see improvements in cholesterol, triglycerides, and blood glucose. Add some regular moderate exercise and the results will be even better. From a strictly medical perspective, there is not much to quibble about, and a body of research supports the benefits of this approach.

Disadvantages: If you're already used to a low-fat diet, you probably don't have a weight problem. For everyone else, maintaining this type of diet requires considerable commitment—indeed, perhaps more than you might be willing to sustain, unless a major heart attack or some other medical crisis precipitated your dietary conversion experience. To shift to daily fare containing less than 10 percent fat represents a rather drastic change for most Americans. Serious makeovers in shopping, food preparation, and eating out need to be learned and practiced. This is one reason why many who launch the Pritikin program do so in a weeklong immersion experience at its Longevity Center. (The calorie-density approach of Robert Pritikin can be eye-opening, but Nutrition Facts labels don't include "calories per pound," and keeping track of these numbers adds another layer to an admittedly challenging task.) While a very low-fat meal, especially one high in fiber, can fill the stomach without a major load of calories, it also won't satisfy hunger nearly as long as a meal with a bit more fat in it. Eating more frequently may result, which may or may not undermine weight-loss efforts, depending on the number of calories involved. In general, many nutrition experts question the wisdom of diets—whether very low fat or very low carbohydrate—that essentially banish an entire class of nutrients. Not all fats are bad for you, and some are essential.

One additional caution: Those who embark on Dr. Ornish's comprehensive program should be aware that his approach to stress management reflects a strong commitment to yoga—not merely as a source of stretching and breathing exercises, but as a comprehensive spiritual worldview.[2] The word *yoga* means "yoke"

[2]See, for example. Dr. Ornish's answer to a question regarding yoga on WebMD at http://my.webmd.com/content/pages/2/3079_1705.htm.

or "union," and the ultimate purpose of yogic practices is to bring about an *experience* of the unity of all things in the universe, a worldview known as monism. While adherents generally claim that yoga is compatible with all religious traditions, its premise and purpose flatly contradict the biblical understanding that God is distinct from His creation (including us), and that He alone is God. Needless to say, it is not necessary to adopt an Eastern religious or mystical worldview in order to lose weight using a low-fat program.

VERY LOW- OR LIMITED-CARBOHYDRATE DIETS

The notion that avoiding or limiting carbohydrates can help you lose weight has been expounded for well over a century, but in the past two decades low-carb diet plans have taken off like a rocket. In case you need convincing, check your neighborhood bookstore or library, where you can find shelves lined with books explaining how to do Atkins, Protein Power, Sugar Busters!, the South Beach Diet, the Carbohydrate Addicts Diet, the Glucose Revolution, the Zone, and a host of others. Many of these have become literal franchises, as the success of an author's first book leads to numerous sequels that provide updated information about the particular plan, new recipes, variations on the diet's basic theme for various groups (kids, adolescents, women, seniors), and so on. The term *Atkins*,

STOP LOOKING FOR THE QUICK FIX

once merely shorthand for the stringent low-carbohydrate program created by Robert C. Atkins, M.D., has
become not only a brand name attached to a variety of
foods but also a part of everyday lingo in phrases such
as "on Atkins," or "Atkins friendly."

If a trip to the bookstore doesn't impress you, check
the labels at your local food store. In the 1980s and
1990s, when fat was widely proclaimed to be the nutritional villain, thousands of "low-fat" and "nonfat" products appeared everywhere in the supermarket. Now food
manufacturers have jumped on the low-carbohydrate
bandwagon, and products claiming to be "low in net
carbs" or "part of your low-carbohydrate lifestyle" are
everywhere.

The low-carb books share some basic assumptions:

1. Carbohydrates—especially sugars and refined
   starches without much fiber—are more rapidly converted to glucose than proteins and fats, causing a
   rise in insulin levels.

2. Insulin not only escorts glucose into cells that need
   it for fuel but also facilitates storage of extra calories
   as fat. It also inhibits mobilization of fat as a source
   of fuel, even when a person is consuming fewer
   calories. Furthermore, a rapid rise in insulin levels
   may result in a drop in blood glucose, causing more
   hunger.

3. All of the advice to eat less fat and more carbohydrates over the past three decades has been mis-
guided and has unintentionally contributed to
America's current epidemic of obesity and diabetes.

4. Limiting your intake of carbohydrates will stop the
glucose-insulin roller coaster and promote weight
loss with much less hunger and hassle than low-fat
diets.

The Atkins diet, introduced in 1972 in the book *Dr.
Atkins' Diet Revolution* and reintroduced in 1992 in *Dr.
Atkins' New Diet Revolution,* takes these assumptions a
step further by recommending very stringent carbohydrate restrictions. During the first two weeks on the
Atkins plan, total carbohydrate intake is to be reduced
to 20 grams per day—the amount in about three cups
of salad—primarily in the form of certain leafy green
vegetables. Sugars and starchy carbohydrates such as
white bread, potatoes, white rice, and pasta from
refined grains are banished more or less indefinitely.
Larger quantities of carbohydrates are allowed over
time depending on the progress of weight loss,
although the types to be eaten (including vegetables
and fruits) are carefully regulated according to their
carbohydrate and fiber content. In dramatic contrast to
the very low-fat approaches of Nathan Pritikin and
Dean Ornish, the Atkins dieter partakes freely of protein and fat. Meats (including red meat), fish (including

shellfish), fowl, cheese, eggs, mayonnaise, butter, and olive oil are all given the green light. For overweight Americans who had been told that they would have to give up so many of their favorite rich foods in order to lose weight, Atkins' regimen sounded like a dream come true.

The paradox of eating rich foods in order to lose weight is explained by a couple of important survival mechanisms. With so little carbohydrate available to serve as fuel, the body taps into its stores of glycogen—the quick-release fuel that we store in limited amounts in muscle and the liver.

Depending on activity levels, glycogen will become depleted within a couple of days, after which the body will begin generating glucose directly from fat. This process releases chemical compounds called ketones into the blood, creating a condition called ketosis (which, by the way, also develops during starvation or an extended fast). Ketosis has the effect of suppressing appetite—a biochemical mercy when no food is available—thus theoretically preventing the Atkins dieter from overdoing the rich foods.

When Atkins' first book appeared in 1972, it was greeted with scorn from the nutritional and medical establishments, which condemned it as dangerous and ineffective. His 1992 follow-up was similarly criticized but sold millions of copies. Critics attributed all weight loss solely to water eliminated from the body when glycogen stores were burned. However, this only accounts for a few pounds and could not explain more substantial weight losses—fifty pounds and beyond—experienced by a number of Atkins dieters. Critics described prolonged ketosis as dangerous, and warnings abounded that the diet's substantial protein intake would overwork or otherwise harm the kidneys. But other than producing a unique breath aroma, ketosis is a physiological adaptation rather than a true disease state (unlike ketoacidosis, an entirely different and very serious condition that can occur among type 1 diabetics—those who are unable to make enough insulin and must take injections to survive). Furthermore, Atkins repeatedly challenged his critics to document a single case in which his diet had actually caused kidney disease or failure. No such cases have made medical headlines, although it should be noted that people who already have impaired kidney function do need to regulate protein intake.

Few if any of the other popular low-carb diets restrict carbohydrates as severely as the Atkins program, but each puts its own variation on what is essentially the same theme. Most have received a chilly reception from mainstream organizations such as the American Dietetic Association and an initial shrug from doctors in everyday practice who typically have little time to sift through the avalanche of these books and programs. So why have these plans sold millions of books, established a growing cultural niche, and even earned some cautious recommendations from physicians?

A reasonable theory. Unlike many fad and crackpot diets that have come and gone over the years, the basic theory of the low- or controlled-carbohydrate plans actually makes some physiological sense. Concepts such as the glycemic index, insulin resistance, and the role of insulin in storing fat aren't bizarre or imaginary. *However:* In order to entice and energize readers, the popular low-carb books tend to oversimplify and over-sell their ideas. The interplay of food, glucose, insulin, hunger, cravings, weight gain, and weight loss is more complex than the picture painted by most of these books. Indeed, much research is underway to clarify these intricate mechanisms.

Unimpressive results from low-fat diets. "Eat less fat" was the dominant advice from nutritional experts (and even doctors) for decades, and yet the nation (including those doctors' patients) not only failed to lose weight but actually got fatter. *However:* Much of the "eat less fat" advice was too vague, such that many overweight people shifted to nonfat sweet and starchy/refined grain foods. Indeed, one of the few points of agreement between low-fat and low-carb advocates is that these foods should be significantly restricted.

More appealing food. Meats, eggs, butter, and

cheese are agreeable to Western palates, so sticking with the plan may be easier—at least for a while. *However:* The stricter the ban on carbohydrates, the harder it is to hang on for the long haul. Eventually most people become weary of avoiding foods such as bread, potatoes, and pasta that they enjoyed for years.

Encouraging results. Many physicians (including Arthur Agatston, M.D., the Florida cardiologist who devised the South Beach Diet) gave low-carb diets a more serious look when some of their patients actually succeeded in losing weight while following them. In 2003, studies began to appear in respectable medical journals demonstrating that in controlled experimental conditions people on low-carbohydrate diets (including ketosis-inducing versions) were more successful at losing weight than those on the typical low-fat diets that had been recommended by mainstream health organizations for decades. Furthermore, weight loss on the low-carb diet resulted in lower cholesterol and triglyceride levels, much to the chagrin of those who had argued that the abundant fat in Atkins and similar diets would have the opposite effect. *However:* While low-carb diets have performed better than low-fat diets in some research studies for periods of about six months, over longer time frames (one year or more) the differences become less obvious. There are no doubt many reasons for this, but an obvious one was already mentioned in connection with both low-carb and low-fat diets: The more restrictive the plan, the less likely a person will stay with it for the long haul.

Should you follow a low- or controlled-carbohydrate diet if you are trying to lose weight? This type of approach may be useful if you have type 2 diabetes because with this condition you're definitely better off limiting the fluctuations in glucose and insulin levels that arise from sugary and starchy foods. Also, many who have struggled with hunger on low-fat diets may experience more success with a controlled-carbohydrate approach. However, you should note the following cautions:

1. The approach you choose should not exclude or strictly limit fruits and vegetables (with the exception of potatoes) for an extended period of time. This is the one area in which tightly controlled low-carbohydrate plans may stray from nutritional common sense. If you are being told to avoid the produce section in order to maintain your low-carb lifestyle, you need to find a different plan.

2. You do not need to spend a lot of time (or any time) in ketosis to lose weight. The Atkins plan involves an extended initial period of ketosis brought on by extremely limited carbohydrate intake. The South Beach Diet proposes a two-week induction period with similar limitations and then shifts to a more liberal carbohydrate intake from fruits and vegetables.

The Zone diet is less restrictive than either of these, proposing that an ideal dietary blend (which helps put one "in the Zone" of optimal health and personal performance) is 30 percent protein, 30 percent fat, and 40 percent carbohydrate. (Zone authors Barry Sears, Ph.D., and Bill Lawren resist classifying their approach as a low-carb diet. However, like the low-carb plans described in this section, their underlying premise is that the benefits of being "in the Zone" derive largely from controlling the flow of glucose and insulin.)

3. Maintaining a low-carbohydrate diet is not a license to ignore portions, the fat content of foods, exercise, or the other important components of managing weight.

"MIDDLE OF THE ROAD" OR LIFESTYLE APPROACHES

These encompass the weight-loss advice you're likely to get from:

- Mainstream professional and academic organizations, such as the American Dietetic Association, the American Heart Association, the American Medical Association, the American Academy of Family Physicians, the Institute of Medicine, Mayo Clinic, and Tufts University Friedman School of Nutrition Science and Policy
- Commercial weight-loss programs such as Weight Watchers or Jenny Craig
- Books such as *Eat, Drink, and Be Healthy*, by Walter C.

Willett, M.D., of Harvard Medical School; *The Ultimate Weight Solution* by Phillip McGraw, Ph.D., (TV's "Dr. Phil"); and *The Tufts University Guide to Total Nutrition*
• Agencies of the federal government such as the Centers for Disease Control and Prevention, the National Institutes of Health, the Food and Drug Administration, and the U.S. Department of Agriculture

You won't get a lot of surprises, magic formulas, or breakthrough revelations about food from these sources. Not all of these are precisely aligned in their approach, but for the most part you'll hear a lot of commonsense advice: decrease your caloric intake and portions, increase exercise, cut the sugar, limit fat to 20 to 30 percent of total calories, eat lots of fruits and veg-etables, and so on.

Advantages: These resources avoid the extremes, the fads, and the weird ideas that waste time, money, and even health. They are committed to solid research and conservative recommendations. If you spend much time with them, you are likely to pick up ideas and even inspiration that will help you lose weight and keep it off.

Disadvantages: The only potential drawback is the "familiarity breeds contempt" problem: You may think, *This is the "same old same old." I've heard it all before, and it didn't work for me.* This is a losing (and we don't mean weight) mind-set, much like avoiding church because you tell yourself, *I've heard it all before.* If you have a long-standing weight problem, you may be particularly vulnerable to the lure of the latest quick fix, when in fact what you need most is to figure out how to make the more reasonable advice work in daily life.

4

THE SECOND KEY: ASSEMBLE YOUR SUPPORT TEAM

If you have a long way to go on the road to weight loss, and especially if you've had a long way to go for a long time, you shouldn't be traveling alone. Breaking loose from tobacco, alcohol, and drug addiction nearly always requires the support of others. In some ways a major weight problem is an even tougher challenge, because there is no way to be abstinent from food. You must interact with it and deal with the physiological and emotional impact of food in your life for months while you are losing weight and for the rest of your life thereafter.

You already know that this is an uphill battle. You want to make healthy eating choices, but your impulses, emotions, and most of the culture push you in the opposite direction. Though you might hope otherwise, you have probably figured out that there isn't a quick fix available now or in the foreseeable future. (Even surgery, for those who are candidates, is such a significant event that counseling and ongoing support, both before and afterward, are very important.) You need teammates and supporters for accountability, encouragement, and even inspiration. This is not a job for a lone ranger.

While each person's circumstances will differ, there are several basic sources of support that you should be thinking about:

God. Acknowledging our dependence on Him for every heartbeat, let alone for success in a chronic struggle such as this, is the beginning of wisdom. Furthermore, if your eating patterns involve compulsive behaviors such as binges or addictions to certain foods, you will need to address the spiritual implications of this type of slavery sooner or later. One of these is acknowledging that a material object (in this case, food) may be displacing God, satisfying needs and forging emotional bonds that rightly should belong to Him alone. Another has long been known to those in Alcoholics Anonymous and other 12-step programs: realizing that we are powerless to manage the addiction (whatever it is), and that we must turn the reins of our lives over to God *daily* in order to do so.

A teammate. One of the best resources you can find for this project will be someone who will cheer you on, hold you accountable in a spirit of love and respect, or (better yet) walk the journey with you. If this person happens to be your spouse and the support is genuine, your likelihood of success will be greatly enhanced. If your spouse isn't interested in volunteering for this role, don't let that deter you, but rather look for another family member or a friend who will walk with you. Caution: If you are making significant changes in your eating habits, you may also have to deal with people, including one or more in your own family, whose words and deeds undermine your efforts.

A class or commercial weight-loss program. In most communities you can find classes or other group programs in a variety of settings: hospitals, churches, community colleges, physicians' offices, a local mall. You should exercise some care before joining one of these, however, in order to avoid exchanging a chunk of your time and money for a lot of frustration. We'll discuss these programs in more detail later in this chapter.

A dietitian. *I've been eating less and exercising more for three months, and the scale hasn't budged. What am I doing wrong?* If you're truly stuck in the process of losing weight, one or more troubleshooting visits with a dietitian can be time very well spent. Of course, you don't have to be at an impasse to seek this type of consultation. If you have a challenging medical or physical problem—you've just had a heart attack or you're newly diagnosed with diabetes or your kidneys aren't functioning properly, for example—you would be wise to have ongoing input from a dietitian. Some or all of your visits may be covered by medical insurance (especially if they are recommended by your physician). Like a private lesson or consultation in any field from skiing to financial planning, you pay extra for personal attention. And like any of those fields, how much you benefit will depend both on the skill of the consultant and your readiness for his or her input.

A support group. Here the emphasis is on interacting with others who are dealing with the same struggle, rather than on hearing instruction from an expert. This may occur informally among friends; within the setting of a church, clinic, or hospital; or under the auspices of groups such as Take Off Pounds Sensibly (TOPS) or Overeaters Anonymous (OA). This is especially important if you need help with compulsive, out-of-control eating patterns. Many churches are now involved in ministries such as Celebrate Recovery that deal not only with alcohol and drugs, but with all forms of compulsions and addictions.

A counselor. Whether you have been waging a long-term battle with significant obesity or have been struggling to maintain your weight, you need to address the emotional issues in your life—especially those that provoke overeating as a form of comfort or self-medication. A trained counselor can help you gain insight and offer strategies that might take much longer to figure out on your own. Some have special training in handling food-related issues, although such expertise is not mandatory for a counselor to provide useful and compassionate help with a weight problem.

MEETING WITH YOUR DOCTOR

At your next medical evaluation, it's important to ask your doctor if you have any health problems that are related to your weight. If you ask *that* question, your doctor will think that you are very astute and hopefully will investigate several factors:

- your actual height, weight, and body mass index (BMI), as well as their trend over the last several years (if your doctor has records extending back that far)
- your blood pressure
- your lipids: cholesterol (total, HDL—high-density lipoproteins or "good" cholesterol—and LDL—low-density lipoproteins or "bad" cholesterol) and triglycerides
- your fasting blood glucose (blood sugar) level, which, if elevated, may lead your doctor to recommend a glucose tolerance test
- any symptoms that might suggest a medical problem aggravated by weight, including chest pain or pressure, shortness of breath, daytime drowsiness, fluid retention, irregular menses, or sore joints (especially knees and hips)
- an electrocardiogram, stress test, or other heart-related studies if you have worrisome chest symptoms or are contemplating vigorous exercise
- any medical problems that might be contributing to your weight problem, such as hypothyroidism or polycystic ovary syndrome

EVALUATING MEDICATIONS AND SUPPLEMENTS

Because losing weight is so often a difficult and demanding process, nearly everyone with this problem has longed for a magic bullet that would

- drastically reduce the appetite,
- reduce or block the absorption of fat or starch,
- rev up metabolism,
- selectively "burn" fat, or
- do all of the above.

The ideal concoction would work without our having to make different choices about food and exercise. Ideally, it would work indefinitely—even during sleep. It also would be completely safe, all natural, and affordable. While we're at it, it would also generate boundless energy, reverse the aging process, and enhance our sex life.

Sound familiar? You have no doubt heard of, and perhaps tried, products that have claimed to do all of this and more. Creative entrepreneurs have utilized all sorts of electrical, magnetic, and mechanical contraptions, not to mention patches, creams, wraps, and shoe inserts, to separate the overweight from their money (but not their extra pounds) and have often made them miserable in the process.

Here's an important bottom line: *At the present time, no nonprescription drug or supplement has been shown to be safe and effective for inducing significant long-term weight loss.* Current federal law allows thousands of nonprescription products to be advertised with all sorts of impressive claims, as long as none of them involve treating a specific disease. Unfortunately, none are evaluated by the Food and Drug Administration (FDA) for safety or effectiveness, although the Federal Trade Commission (FTC) may issue warnings to distributors if they are making blatantly misleading statements about their products. Furthermore, a product will be taken off the market only if it is found to be harmful.

This in fact occurred with ephedra, a stimulant found in many weight-loss aids (often in the form of the herb *ma huang*) that has been linked to irregular heart rhythm, high blood pressure, stroke, seizures, and even death. In 2004, the FDA prohibited the sale of supplements containing ephedra, although a few may still be in circulation. Another nonprescription drug that was banned by the FDA is phenyl-propanolamine (or PPA), once found both in cold tablets and in diet aids such as Dexatrim and AcuTrim. PPA raised blood pressure and pulse rate too often to be considered safe, and it was even associated with hemorrhagic (bleeding) strokes.

Unfortunately, as obesity has become more widespread in the United States, hundreds of marketers have taken advantage of the opportunity to make some serious cash by offering quick and easy cures to the frustrated and desperate. There are in fact so many weight-loss products lining the shelves and advertised on radio, TV, and especially the Internet that it would be impossible to list even a fraction of them, let alone analyze them. Instead, we will list a number of red-flag claims that are literally too good to be true and that virtually guarantee that a product isn't worth your hard-earned money. Many are a variation on the magic-bullet wish list we included at the beginning of this section:

- You'll lose two or more pounds every week for several weeks, no matter what you eat and without exercise. *Reality check:* This is the most common—and the least truthful—claim made for weight-loss products. Unfortunately, this promise is a biological fantasy.
- The product, with or without additional calorie restriction, will cause pounds to "melt away" at spectacular rates (such as a pound per day) for several weeks. *Reality check:* Those who cut their calorie intake significantly will burn glycogen for fuel, and this can result in the loss of several pounds of fluid. It's encouraging, but it isn't fat. Since a pound of fat represents 3,500 stored calories, to lose a pound of fat in one day would require one to eat nothing while exercising like a lumberjack from dawn until dusk. It doesn't happen.
- The weight you lose will be permanent. The pounds will stay off, even if you stop using the product. *Reality check:* You can in fact keep the weight off after stopping the product—by maintaining different eating and exercise habits. In other words, you really didn't need the product in the first place.

- The product will prevent the absorption of fat, resulting in substantial weight loss. *Reality check:* You can lose a modest amount of weight with Xenical, a prescription drug that interferes with fat absorption, but it's hardly a free ride. The only people who lose substantial pounds by failing to absorb nutrients are those with diseases known as malabsorption syndromes, which can pose a serious threat to health.
- The product will produce dramatic results for anyone who uses it. *Reality check:* When you're talking about any dietary program, medication, or supplement, remember this important phrase: "Results may vary." Nothing works for everyone.
- Wearing the product or rubbing it on the skin leads to substantial weight loss. *Reality check:* There is no medical evidence, or even a rational explanation, to support this type of claim, which is the nutritional equivalent of Bigfoot, Elvis sightings, and the tooth fairy.
- The product is marketed using testimonials. *Reality check:* This is the least reliable measure of a product's effectiveness. Talk is cheap, and it can easily be purchased by the marketer. Scientifically valid proof that a product is safe and effective requires careful, controlled studies involving large numbers of people.
- The product contains a formula that is unique, superior to anything on the market, and not available anywhere else. *Reality check:* In psychiatry such claims would be called delusions of grandeur. Steer clear of any practitioner who offers a treatment or product that is "the only one of its kind," or who implies that "everyone is wrong but me."

- The product was developed by a leading expert in the field of nutrition. *Reality check:* There are countless self-proclaimed experts in nutrition. The professionals who are truly respected in this field aren't hawking products on the Internet.

What about prescription medications? Can your doctor prescribe a medication that will help you jump-start a diet plan? Mainstream medical thinking has shifted from viewing obesity as a character flaw to treating it as a significant disorder with important health consequences. Furthermore, pharmaceutical manufacturers are well aware that any product that *really* helps people lose excess weight, and does it safely, will be a literal gold mine. As a result, currently a number of promising medications are slowly wending their way through the laborious and expensive development-and-testing process before getting the FDA's green light to enter the marketplace. (This is drastically different from the unregulated environment in which nonprescription drugs are unleashed upon the public.)

At the time of this book's writing, several medications are available at your local pharmacy that might enhance the results of dietary and exercise efforts, but they are hardly miracle drugs that will zap your appetite or melt away the fat. At best they may contribute to a 5 to 10 percent weight loss over the course of several months. This may not seem spectacular, but it could actually make a significant difference in your cholesterol, triglyceride, or blood glucose levels. This would please your doctor, even if it didn't drastically alter what you see in the mirror.

GETTING THE MOST FROM A NUTRITION PROGRAM OR A WEIGHT-LOSS CONSULTANT

You've decided that it's time to get some help losing weight. Should you join Weight Watchers, try Jenny Craig, see a dietitian, or check out a local weight-loss clinic that just opened? Here's the bottom line first: Think and evaluate carefully *before* you spend your time and money on a program, a dietitian, a nutrition-ist, or other weight-loss consultant. What specifically should you be thinking about?

Why am I doing this?
Some good reasons to begin such a program are to establish some basic structure for your food choices and a track to run on for the long haul, as well as to receive troubleshooting, insight, accountability, and encouragement.

Some bad reasons are the desire for a quick fix, a magic formula, rapid weight loss, and a radical and restrictive diet, or simply to achieve short-term goals.

The good reasons involve a mind-set that *you,* not someone else, are ultimately in charge and responsible for your health, and that whatever you do must work for the rest of your life. The program or the individual is providing advice and expertise to assist you in the process. The bad reasons involve a passive but often desperate mind-set: *Do something, anything, to me or for me so that I will lose weight without having to address my daily choices.* They also reflect unrealistic expectations and reliance on exotic food formulas or (worse) expensive supplements, rather than an understanding of why some foods are better than others and what behaviors contribute to weight gain.

What are the components of the program?
Don't sign up for any program without knowing exactly what is included—and what you'll be expected to pay for.

Information. Do you just get a list of dos and don'ts, or does the program provide ongoing *education* about nutrition, foods, meal preparation, and managing your own behavior? Learning to eat well is an important long-term life skill, and the more you know, the more likely you are to make better decisions in the long run. You shouldn't settle for a no-brainer approach to weight loss.

Diet plans. What exactly is the approach to food while you're losing weight? Is the focus on reduced calories, very low calories, low fat, low carb, high protein, food combining, or some other approach? If the plan is extreme (for example, no fats, no carbohydrates, or just fruits, etc.) or far removed from what you're used to eating, it may seem easier to follow . . . at first. It's like starting a really tight, no-frills budget: There's less to think about, and making a decisive change can feel downright energizing. *Hey, I'm really doing something!* If the eating plan is highly restrictive and doesn't include your usual comfort foods, you'll tend to eat simply to quell hunger and not for pleasure, so the pounds will indeed disappear. This is why virtually any diet plan will work—for a while. But as time passes and the novelty wears off, the old foods will begin to sing their siren song. If the plan doesn't have a contingency plan for your previous habits other than "just say no," in a moment of weakness it may get the heave-ho, along with the money you spent on it.

Your food or their food? Some commercial plans offer to supply some or all of your food, prepared, prepackaged, and ready to eat. The advantage of this is that you don't have to do a lot of thinking or preparation, and as long as you carefully follow the program's guidelines, you'll probably lose weight. Also, eating such prepared foods may give you an idea of what reasonable portions of food actually look like. However, such a plan will be more expensive than preparing your own food, and if you don't care for the program's bill of fare, you'll be tempted to cheat. If you're doing prepackaged foods and hope to succeed, your family will have to fend for themselves in the kitchen; it takes nerves of steel to prepare food for others that you're not supposed to eat. Also, since you're not likely to buy from this "store" for the rest of your life, it's often difficult to make the transition from their food to normal food.

Very little food. Some programs give you "substitute meals"—usually some form of powdered concoction that you stir into cold water and drink like a milk shake (only it's not as enjoyable)—in place of one or two regular meals. (Products such as Slim·Fast that serve this purpose are also available at the store; you don't need to join a program to use them.) Very low-calorie diets (sometimes known as protein-sparing fasts) drop daily calorie intake to no more than 800 calories, an approach that should only be undertaken under close medical supervision, if ever. As we said earlier, the more restricted eating plans may be more efficient at helping you lose weight in the short run, but you must eventually address a crucial question: *What am I going to do for the rest of my life?* If you go back to the same eating habits, guess what? The pounds you worked so hard to lose will come back, and they may bring a few friends with them.

Medications, shots, or supplements. Beware—if a program offers diet pills or special injections that will "melt off the fat," your chances of long-term success are poor, and you can count on shelling out a fair amount of money that would be better spent elsewhere (such as on fresh vegetables and fruit).

Who's running the program, and what are their credentials?

You should review this information before any money changes hands. Ideally, a comprehensive program utilizes the services of one or more physicians, registered dietitians, psychologists/counselors, and physical therapists or trainers, all of whom have special expertise in medicine, nutrition, behavior modification, and exercise as they relate to weight loss. Often such programs are formally affiliated with well-established institutions such as universities, regional medical centers, or even local hospitals. At the other end of the spectrum are storefront clinics run by a self-proclaimed expert with little or no formal training.

Beware: Many "nutritionists" with eccentric or even bizarre notions of dietary health offer worthless but often costly tests that are supposed to determine your individual nutrient needs and deficiencies. Worse yet, they frequently have shelves of expensive vitamins and supplements that they promise will correct whatever is wrong, to the tune of one or two hundred dollars per month, or even more.

Before starting a program, find out what type of formal training the staff members have had. This may be easier said than done. Your own physician, for example, may not have much expertise on this subject. Unfortunately, there is no shortage of bogus nutritional schools and "professional" organizations willing to grant degrees or other credentials to anyone who signs up and pays a fee. Furthermore, while it is possible for any health professional (or for that matter a layperson) to gain solid knowledge of nutrition and weight-management techniques through personal study and continuing education courses, the recognized experts in the field are registered dietitians (R.D.'s).

The person with an R.D. credential has earned at least a bachelor's degree from an accredited university or college, with coursework approved by the American Dietetic Association's accrediting organization, the Commission on Accreditation for Dietetics Education (CADE); completed a supervised practice program, usually six to twelve months in length, at a CADE-accredited health-care facility, community agency, or food-service corporation; passed a national examination administered by the Commission on Dietetic Registration (CDR), which also awards credentials for dietetic technicians as well as specialists in pediatric nutrition and renal nutrition; and maintained the R.D. credential through ongoing professional education.

For an individual consultation, a registered dietitian is nearly always the best bet.

What kinds of long-term results is the program achieving?

Do any studies or statistics back up the program's claims? Remember—the fact that many clients are able to lose several pounds over the first few weeks may sound impressive, but how many have been able to maintain substantial weight loss over six months, a year, or longer?

How much is it going to cost?

You may be desperate to lose weight and impressed by what you've heard, but don't overlook the M word: money. Most programs charge a basic fee to participate, and then you pay extra for food, meal substitutes, medications (if a physician in the program prescribes them), supplements, vitamins, or other services such as lab tests. All of these extras can cost you, so think carefully about what you really need. If the program wants you to get a fasting chemistry and lipid profile but your doctor recently ran the same tests, there may be no need to repeat them right away. Also, your health insurance may cover such tests if ordered by your physician, but not necessarily if they're done by a commercial weight-loss program.

Speaking of insurance, some visits with a registered dietitian or participation in a program (especially one operated from a physician's office, licensed clinic, or hospital) may be at least partially reimbursed by your health plan. Usually this requires an order from your physician, and the dietary consultation or weight-loss program must be tied to a specific medical diagnosis (for example, type 2 diabetes).

Another option is a maximum-impact, multi-disciplinary live-in program in which you turn your focus entirely on weight issues for a specified time, such as one or two weeks. These all-inclusive jump starts are quite expensive, and long-term follow-through is essential to get your money's worth. Otherwise, you know what will happen: It's relatively easy to feel inspired and do the right thing when you're immersed in a culture of healthy eating and the food is carefully regimented. But what happens when you return to your own home and job? You need some new coping skills and someone to call if you're having trouble staying the course, or your investment may be squandered.

5

THE THIRD KEY: BEGIN MAKING SMARTER FOOD CHOICES

This is perhaps the most confusing part of a weight-loss project, because there are so many contradictory views on what constitutes the "right" foods both for weight loss and for general nutrition. The following are some basic principles of healthy eating:

1. **Phase out the sugary foods.** Soft drinks (the nondiet variety), cookies, cakes, candies, pastries, and other sugary foods are the classic empty calories that need to be eaten sparingly, or phased out of your life entirely. This is one idea that both low-fat and low-carb advocates agree upon.

2. **Gravitate toward whole-grain foods rather than those made from refined or processed grains**. For many people, especially those with type 2 diabetes, limiting those foods (as well as sugars) that are rapidly converted into glucose may lead to more

effective weight loss. Whole-grain foods also contain more valuable nutrients, vitamins, and fiber.

3. **Eat five to nine servings of fruits and vegetables (not counting potatoes) every day.** You need to think beyond the lettuce in your salad, by the way, and sample the rainbow of fruit and vegetable colors—green, yellow, red, orange, white, and even blue. Spend more time in the produce section or at a local farmer's market and less in the meat section.

4. **Eat lean meats in modest portions**—three to four ounces, about the size of a deck of cards—and think baked, broiled, or grilled rather than deep fried.

5. **Keep an eye on the cholesterol content of foods.** Cholesterol itself doesn't contribute to excess weight, but it tends to come along for the ride in many calorie-dense foods that do. (Important reminder: If you are overweight and a blood test shows that you have a high level of cholesterol, losing excess weight will lower the cholesterol level much more efficiently than simply limiting the amount of cholesterol you eat.)

6. **Gravitate to the "good" fats.** These are the monounsaturated fats contained in olive and canola oils, as well as in cold-water-dwelling fish. When you can, substitute olive oil for butter or margarine in your food preparation.

Here's an important take-home message: *No single approach, formula, or plan for weight loss can work for every person.* You must learn basic, sound nutritional concepts and then adapt them to your (and your family's) unique circumstances, lifestyle, likes, and dislikes. This may sound like we're stating the obvious, but in the search for surefire formulas it's easy to miss the obvious: *If your approach to losing weight doesn't work for you, it isn't going to work at all.*

EAT LESS (AND EAT MORE SLOWLY)

This obvious point is so often overlooked in the frantic search for the secret to losing weight. Whether you gravitate toward a plan that is low fat, low carb, both, or neither, you will need to deal with this part of the equation. If you're overweight and staying overweight (or getting more overweight with each passing year), guess what? Over the long haul, whatever you're eating contains more calories than your body needs. Keep in mind some basic arithmetic: A pound of stored fat represents an extra 3,500 calories of energy. That means an excess of only 100 calories per day—what you'll find in about eight ounces of your favorite nondiet soft drink—will add ten pounds to your body in a year. The good news is that consistent small-scale reductions will also pay off if you give them enough time.

Like it or not, even if you're eating smarter (that is, choosing better quality food) it is very difficult to lose weight without addressing the amount of food you consume every day. Obviously, downsizing the amount of food we eat is easier said than done when so much is available everywhere we turn. So here's a top-ten list to help you adjust the amount of food you eat.

1. **Eat when you're hungry—and stop when you're not.** This is a profoundly simple idea, but we're so used to eating for every possible reason that this may prove harder than it sounds. Before you start eating, or before the next bite, get in the habit of asking yourself, *Am I (still) hungry?* You may be surprised at how often the answer is *Not really,* at which point you need to ask, *So why am I reaching for something to put in my mouth?* If the answer is that you're upset, bored, or trying to relax, then ask yourself if there are other ways to solve that problem, even if they may not seem as quick and effective as your favorite food. If the answer is, *I'm enjoying this, and I don't feel like stopping,* then at least slow down (see number 3). Many people dread embarking on a weight-loss effort because they anticipate being hungry and miserable day and night. Here's a news flash—*you do not need to go hungry in order to lose weight.* In fact, you're more likely to yield to the worst food temptations if you're famished. If you're actually feeling hungry, you should eat something—but of course *what* and *how much* will be the critical issues.

By the way, most of us eat so often that we don't know the difference between real hunger and every other vague uneasiness that seems to respond to food. If you have any doubt, try skipping one or two meals and note how you feel. Then as an experiment, see how little food it takes to end that sensation.

2. **Stop eating when you're satisfied, but before you're really full.** We all enjoy eating a traditional Thanksgiving dinner, but how often have you left the table feeling more stuffed than the turkey? That bloated, heavy, drowsy sensation really isn't very pleasant, nor are the heartburn and gas that may join the party a little later. Unfortunately, eating a complete dinner at many restaurants—or perhaps at your dining-room table—will bring on the same sensation. In many cultures children are taught to stop eating before they feel full, and we should learn to do likewise. (Hunger will be gone long before you've eaten half of the amount that brings fullness.)

3. **Eat slowly.** If you've ever been interrupted for several minutes after the first few bites of a meal, you may have noticed that you weren't particularly hungry when you sat down again. This is a very important validation of the fact that *whether we eat quickly or slowly, hunger goes away in about the same amount of time.* Think of it another way. After you begin eating, it takes about fifteen to twenty minutes for signals

from the stomach and changes in blood glucose to signal that you're no longer hungry. If you are inhaling your food during that time, you can put away hundreds of calories—and yet be no more satisfied than if you took a fraction of that amount.

If you really enjoy food, eating slowly is the only way to go:

- Put down your utensils between bites.
- After cutting a piece of meat, put the knife down and pick up the fork with the hand that held the knife—then eat the piece of meat. (This avoids the rapid-fire fork-to-mouth routine.)
- Take smaller bites.
- Thoroughly chew, and savor the taste and texture of each mouthful.
- Pause between bites. If you're with others, enjoy the conversation. If everyone is too busy eating to talk, start some conversation so that *they'll* slow down. (If a TV is the yammering "guest" at your meal, by all means turn it off.) A shared meal at which no one is talking is a wasted opportunity. If you're eating alone, stop and give thanks for every bite.

4. **Think differently about portions (part 1).** Here's the simplest, cheapest, most surefire weight-loss program on the planet, and it involves only three basic steps:
   - Put whatever you're used to eating at a given meal on your plate.
   - Take half of it away.

- Eat what remains slowly enough to last as long as your regular portions.

Okay, so this advice was a little tongue-in-cheek, but not entirely. Assuming that you don't need a complete overhaul of your food choices, if you're overweight and not making any progress, then whatever you're eating is sustaining (or building) your current weight. Removing half of your usual portions would be a pretty drastic change, but it would certainly work. Taking away a quarter or a third of your typical portions will almost certainly work over time, assuming you stick with it.

5. **Think differently about portions (part 2).** Here's another cheap and simple weight-loss program, also a little tongue-in-cheek:
    - Find a thin person your age and gender who appears to enjoy life and good health.
    - Observe carefully what and how much that person eats.
    - Go and do likewise.

There will of course be differences between you in genetics and activity level, but don't be surprised if you also find some important differences between the sizes of the portions you consume. Forget about sixteen-ounce steaks and baked potatoes the size of a football. Think instead about adopting some of the following portion sizes—none of which require you to use a food scale—for foods that are often sources of runaway calories:

- a piece of lean meat the size of a deck of cards
- a potato the size of a small lightbulb
- a serving of cheese the size of one or two pairs of dice
- a serving of butter the size of one of those dice
- a serving of pasta the size of the mouse that you use with your computer
- a one-cup serving of cereal (one of the good kinds, without all of the added sugar), which is also the amount in one of those individual-sized boxes
- one slice of bread, half a bagel, half an English muffin, or half a bun

Notice that we didn't list serving sizes for foods like broccoli, apples, and celery sticks. The vast majority of vegetables and fruits are part of the solution rather than part of the problem, unless they're swimming in rich sauces or syrups.

6. **Think differently about portions (part 3).** Here's our third and final cheap and simple weight-loss plan:
   - Instead of the typical dinner plate, use a salad plate to hold your usual fare. (You can have another salad plate for the salad.)
   - Don't eat any more than you can fit on that plate—no stacking allowed—and no going back for seconds.
   - Take your sweet time eating your meal.

Remember the good old days when you would receive an actual hot meal on a long airline flight? Remember the tiny salad and the little rectangular container that held the main course? There wasn't much there, but because it filled the dish completely it always seemed like enough food. If you're trying to reduce portions and place some smaller servings on your old dinner plate, all of that open space may look alarming. *Is that all I get??* Put it on a smaller plate, however, and your brain will adjust its perception and your emotions.

7. **Avoid random or nonpurposeful eating.** There are all sorts of occasions when we eat not because we're hungry or even to comfort ourselves (more on that later), but just because the food happens to appear before us. A lot of people have trouble with this at the workplace: Someone has a birthday or a coworker brings leftovers from a party at home, and suddenly there's an array of our favorite snack foods on the counter as we pass by. If it's something we like, it's all too easy to reach for it without thinking, an automatic reflex between brain, arm, and mouth. It takes some effort, but it's critical to ask yourself the all-important questions: (1) *Am I actually hungry?* (2) *If I am actually hungry, is this plateful of cake/cookies/chips the best way to relieve my hunger?*

If you're an autopilot eater, you must create an environment at home that reduces the likelihood of this behavior. It's very simple: When you're done eating, put *all* of the food away. You can consider making an exception for a bowl of fruit, especially if you're trying to reprogram your household to enjoy more nutritious snacks. Some important variations on this theme:

- **The big one: eating in front of the TV.** This spells trouble in three ways. First, while engrossed in a program or a movie you can easily lose track of what you're eating and consume a tremendous quantity of food—especially those snacks that you don't actually put on a plate but rather pull out of a bag or box one after another. Second, TV watching is a sedentary (i.e., sitting or lying down) rather than active pastime. More hours in front of the tube mean fewer hours moving muscle. *This is especially important for children and adolescents,* for whom TV watching is frequently associated with excessive weight. Third, you're likely to see enticing ads for all kinds of food.

  Taming the TV and snacking monster may be a challenge, especially if this habit is entrenched in your (and your family's) life. It's all about taking charge: *You* decide how much and what you're going to watch, rather than simply turning the set on and mindlessly surfing through 150 channels. If there's going to be food in the TV room, *you* decide ahead of time what and how much. Don't just bring boxes, bags, and bowls of stuff to graze on. Another interesting option is to propose that anyone watching TV, including you, does some sort of exercise—aerobic, strength training, or stretching—at the same time. This not only solves the snacking problem but also improves everyone's physical condition and tends to cut the number of hours spent in front of the tube.

- **Eating at sporting events and movies.** Once again, a little planning can save you hundreds of excess calories, not to mention a wad of cash. For one thing, don't come to the game or movie hungry. If the venue allows it, bring some healthier snacks of your own, such as fruit or sticks of carrots or celery. If not, look for smaller sizes or split larger quantities among two or more people. Consider getting ice water instead of a soft drink, and hold the butter on the popcorn. And as always, ask the important question: *Am I still hungry?*

- **Eating during other activities.** Many weight-loss programs advise that when you are at home, you should eat only from one (modest-sized) plate, in one room, doing absolutely nothing else. If you want a snack, fine—just measure out a reasonable portion on your special plate, and then eat it at your kitchen or dining-room table without watching TV, reading, studying, or doing anything else. (Obviously, having a conversation with another person is okay—otherwise, eating becomes like sharing a trough in the barn.) In general this is a good idea for limiting random, unconscious eating, but with one exception. If you're eating an actual meal (as opposed to a snack) by yourself, reading may help you *take your time* with it, as long as you keep track of your hunger/fullness status.

8. **Get comfortable leaving food behind.** Many of us are driven by the insane notion that we are obliged to finish whatever food appears on our plate. This may arise from exhortations during childhood to "Join the clean-plate club" or "Remember that people are starving in Africa," or messages from Mom or Grandma that preparing food is a gesture of love and

eating it is a way of saying thank you. How many times have we kept eating (especially in a restaurant and often long after being full) because we didn't want food to go to waste? If the only two destinations for that food are the trash bin or the bulging fat stores in our body, which is the better place for it to go? "I paid good money for that food," you might protest. But what is the excess fat costing you? And if you're in a restaurant, your server will gladly give you a box or bag to take home the extra for another day.

Very important parenting tip: Don't encourage or exhort kids to eat when they're not hungry, and don't threaten to punish them for not cleaning their plates. There are much healthier ways to influence what they eat.

9. **Be very careful when you eat out.** Enjoying restaurant meals can be both a treat and a trap. Yes, it's nice for special occasions, but all too often we opt for the drive-through, the pizza delivery, or even a complete sit-down meal because we're too rushed or hassled or tired to prepare food ourselves. About 25 percent of American meals are not home cooked, and that's not counting "nuke and serve" foods from the freezer. Not only can this be a drain on the pocketbook, but many restaurants serve up very large portions, whether or not they're designated as

supersized. Here are some suggestions to help draw the line between dining out and pigging out:

- Try to avoid bringing a ravenous appetite to the restaurant. You'll be tempted to order more items than you really need.

- Take your time. The fact that families often go to restaurants because there isn't time to *prepare* a meal doesn't mean that "eating out" has to mean "eat and run." The best restaurant experiences are those in which the meal is an occasion to share good conversation, not to rush through the food. The more expensive fine-dining establishments have this figured out: They tend to serve smaller portions (often exquisitely prepared) at a leisurely pace, leaving you satisfied but not bloated.

- Split entrees. If you and your companion can find something you both like, this will save both money and calories.

- As we just said, you don't have to clean your plate. Stop when you're pleasantly satisfied, and ask to have what remains put in a container to take home.

- Skip dessert or order one for the whole table to share.

- Stay out of fast-food restaurants. Many overweight people can date some of their most dramatic weight gain to a period of time when the pressures of life led to frequent stops at fast-food franchises. The products they serve are carefully engineered to be highly satisfying— indeed, some would argue that they are addictive, especially to young palates whose business they aggressively court. In response to rising criticism about dispensing nutritional junk, the fast-food industry has started to offer some alternatives to the usual burgers and fries, including salads, broiled chicken entrées, and fruit.

But their staple items remain highly processed, calorie dense, and loaded with saturated fat, salt, and sugar.

- If you can't stay out of fast-food restaurants, skip the fries and look for a salad. Avoid supersizing, the marketing ploy that seems like such a bargain but packs huge amounts of extra calories. The only items that get supersized are fries and soft drinks, which you should avoid anyway. Get the kids—and yourselves—milk or water instead of a soft drink.
- Avoid buffets, or at least don't come with a huge appetite. For the person with a weight problem, a buffet line represents a major challenge. Who can resist all of those appealing items, especially when it's all to be had for one price? Even small portions of a dozen different items can result in a calorie pileup. When faced with a buffet meal, follow some of the other guidelines in this section: put your choices on a smaller plate (usually the salad plate), eat slowly, quit before you're full, and don't feel obliged to finish what's on your plate, even though you put it there yourself.

10. **Keep your eyes open for other ideas like these, and for recipes that utilize healthier foods and portions.** No single source of advice, including this book, will address *every* issue you might have related to weight or portions. While you don't want to obsess about what you eat or make food the center of your emotional universe, this is such an important topic that you would be wise to become a lifelong learner.

THE FOURTH KEY: ADOPT HELPFUL ATTITUDES AND HABITS

Throughout this book, we emphasize the principle that weight loss is a gradual but steady process. In order to succeed, there are some key lifestyle patterns that need to be established. In this chapter we will show you how to create habits that help you resist food temptations and ensure that the pounds you work so hard to lose stay away.

IDENTIFY AND ADDRESS YOUR TRIGGERS

Spend some time thinking about the times and circumstances where you become vulnerable to overeating. For example: *At the end of the day, I'm exhausted and my resistance is definitely low. If the kids [or boss or customers] have been pushing me all day, I just need something that will relax me, and nothing works like a quart of ice cream.*

What else could you do at that moment that would distract you until the impulse passes? These alternatives to food need to be realistic, readily available, and capable of bringing you some satisfaction. Your options might include:

- going for a brisk walk
- taking a hot, relaxing bath
- doing some stretches
- praying or contemplating
- cleaning something
- getting rid of some clutter
- venting to a family member or friend
- watching a half hour of an upbeat, cheerful, or otherwise diverting program

My day is wall-to-wall with commitments: work, appointments, errands, church activities, chauffeuring kids, you name it. I don't even have time to nuke something out of the freezer, let alone prepare gourmet meals for myself or anyone else. When I'm hungry I need to grab and go, and fast food is my best friend. If you're a frequent flyer at the drive-through, or you stop at gas-station minimarts to fill your tank more often than the car's, or the take-out crew at the local pizza parlor knows your order and your address as soon as you say your name, you may be blowing too much cash for too many calories. Unfortunately, solving this requires some time and planning. Sometime when you're not going ninety miles per hour, sit down for a few minutes and think about preparing some healthier (and less expensive) food. Pace your intake throughout the day, so you don't become ravenous and head for the nearest vending machine or fast-food emporium. For what you'd save by bypassing the burgers and fries, you could buy an insulated food carrier for work or your car.

Every time the family [or congregation or work group] gathers for some socializing, all we do is eat. I don't want to be a snob or a party pooper, and I don't want to just sit there while everyone else enjoys the feast. Again, a little planning is in order, whether you're going to a birthday party, a church supper, or a corporate banquet:

- Avoid coming with a serious appetite. You'll be less tempted to overindulge.
- If the setting is informal, use the salad-plate approach (page 60) to downsize your meal, especially at a potluck.
- As mentioned earlier, take your time between bites. You can enjoy the meal and make it last as long as everyone else's, without the calories and bloating.
- Focus more on the conversation than the food.

You get the idea. Sometime when you're not rushed, think through your last—and your next—typical week. Recall when the eating got out of control and what prompted it. Then consider how you might avoid the same result next time.

Another instructive approach is to keep a food diary for two weeks. Without adjusting what you normally do to make the diary look respectable, write down *everything* you eat, including snacks. Make note of the time, the place, the type of food, and the amount eaten, as well as whether or not you were hungry, and how you were feeling at the time.

For the quantity, don't get hung up on the exact amount. An estimate based on size ("a steak the size of both hands") will do. More important is to identify the emotion that accompanied the food (happy, sad, bored, frustrated, celebrative, etc.). Getting a grip on how much and how often you eat, and what triggers your desire for food, can be very informative. Many people find that they begin to modify their eating habits just as a result of keeping these notes and becoming more aware of their patterns. In addition, if you seek help from a dietitian, bringing a two-week food diary will make his or her job much easier.

MODIFY YOUR ENVIRONMENT (IN OTHER WORDS, FLEE TEMPTATION)

If you're trying to quit smoking or drinking alcohol, guess what you shouldn't have lying around your house? Cigarettes or alcohol. Similarly, if certain foods are your downfall, then by all means *get them out of sight and out of reach.* If your cupboards are full of cookies and chips and your fridge is bulging with ice cream and soft drinks, your job will be much harder. If these foods are beckoning you from open bowls or boxes, you can count on your weight-loss efforts failing. But if these temptations aren't readily available, you've created a line of defense against impulse eating.

But the kids and my spouse will complain if I don't bring

this stuff home. The short answer is *too bad.* The longer
answers are:

- Junk food isn't doing them any good. If your kitchen is
  full of healthier and more nutritious options, everybody
  wins.
- Are you buying these goodies for them . . . or for you?
- If anyone else in the family is struggling with weight—
  especially one or more children or teenagers—it's
  important to make their environment as temptation-free
  as possible.
- Whether only one person in the family is too heavy or
  everyone could stand to shape up, the family needs to
  work as a team to support (or at least not undermine) the
  weight-loss effort.

Caution: Your efforts to purge the home of
unhealthy, high-calorie snacks would be best done
without becoming a dietary Darth Vader or a food
fascist. Talk with your family about the changes you
(and they) need to make, and get their input. (Mom
and Dad should already be on the same page before
this conversation. If not, any disgruntled children will
quickly divide and conquer to disrupt your efforts.)
You may discover that they're not as attached to these
foods as you thought. Your family may also prefer to
phase in this process over time. For example, if you've
been buying megabags of chips, try an assortment of
individual servings instead. They're not as economical,
but the calorie savings may well be worth it. The same
goes for buying individual, smaller containers of soda

or juice drinks rather than liter- or larger-sized bottles. Consider low-fat, reduced-sugar frozen yogurt rather than ice cream, or some fresh fruit instead of either of these for dessert.

Here are some other areas you need to be thinking about:

- Do you allow (or sneak) food all over the house?
- Do you do a lot of eating in the car?
- Does your workplace seem like an open vending machine?
- Does your route to and from work or your most common errands take you through "franchise row," from which all of your favorite foods call your name?
- Do you buy groceries from a list, or do you wander the aisles picking up whatever looks appealing?

All of these, and no doubt many others as well, are situations that cue you to eat, or at least to think about food, usually when you're not particularly hungry. Smokers who are trying to quit have to deal with this all day long, because so many events—a cup of coffee, a phone call, a ride in the car, and many more— become linked to lighting a cigarette. You can spend a lot of energy trying to uncouple the stimulus (that is, the sight, smell, or even thought of food) from the response (eating). But doing this involves exercising our willpower, which for most of us can fluctuate through the course of the day.

Why make the battle harder than it already is? It's a lot easier and more practical to reduce the number of opportunities for the unwanted behavior. Someone who is trying to stay sober should stay out of cocktail lounges. A man who has problems with Internet pornography should avoid being alone with an online computer. A compulsive shopper shouldn't walk into a mall with a wallet full of credit cards. If you have a weight problem, it only makes sense to take some control of your environment in order to reduce the opportunities for snacking, impulsive eating, or even binging.

ADDRESS THE EMOTIONAL AND SPIRITUAL ISSUES RELATED TO EATING

This is extremely important, because for so many who are overweight or obese, *food is the drug of choice to relieve emotional or even spiritual discomfort*. This is particularly critical if food binges (episodes in which hundreds or even thousands of calories are consumed) are part of your weight problem. Indeed, compulsive behaviors—whether involving eating, smoking, abuse of alcohol or other drugs, shopping, pornography, sex, gambling, you name it—all serve some emotional purpose, most often an immediate reduction of discomfort. These behaviors inevitably have serious, or even lethal, long-term consequences. Yet the most severe pain and suffering may not be enough to override whatever pleasure or relief the substance or behavior provides at the moment.

Wait a minute. I'm not like one of those drug addicts on

the street. I'm behaving responsibly at home, work, and
church, and getting quite a bit accomplished as well.

So noted, and much appreciated. But you can be a
good person and do all of those good things, and still
have a serious weight problem because eating is a form
of release that happens to be legal, easily obtainable,
quickly satisfying in public or in secret, and rarely sin-
gled out in church as a moral issue. Whether a full-
blown compulsion or a quiet release, eating can be a
response to any number of emotional aches and pains:

- the stresses of life, whether minor or monumental
- anxiety, whether short-term or chronic
- frustration over today's events—or all of life
- anger and its chronic cousin, bitterness
- fatigue
- boredom
- loneliness
- depression
- a defense against intimacy or attention from the
  opposite sex

The last item on this list might seem surprising—
doesn't the overweight person long for a sexually
attractive body? Certainly many do, but some women
who have been sexually abused in the past may uncon-
sciously seek protection from further exposure to this
trauma by wrapping themselves in enough fat to ward
off male attention.

Acquiring and maintaining emotional health is a lifelong, multidimensional process. It is also directly con-

nected with spiritual health, because experiencing an intimate, nurturing experience with God plays a foundational role in the way you look at yourself, your life, and the people around you.

If you have a long-standing and seemingly unmanageable weight problem, it is unlikely that you will solve it merely by adjusting the types and amounts of food you eat. Even if you feel that any emotional issues are the result rather than the cause of the weight, it is essential that you begin to deal with them—and to do some exploring of underlying currents as well. This may involve individual counseling, a small group within your church in which you feel safe dealing with difficult and personal subjects, or a support group specifically focused on weight issues, such as Overeaters Anonymous.

GIVE THIS PROJECT THE TIME AND ATTENTION IT DESERVES

If you get nothing else from this segment, take this thought home: If you have a significant weight problem, and especially if you have fought a losing battle for years, don't sell yourself short by taking a random stab at it now and again. Don't pursue the quick fixes and the magic formulas and the miracle supplements. They'll waste your time and money, and they can make your problem worse if your weight yo-yos up and down with each passing fad. It takes time to learn the basics of nutrition, to become a smarter shopper, to try new and healthier recipes, to figure out what you're preparing for dinner tomorrow rather than hitting the drive-through, to exercise, to work on your emotional issues, to meet with health professionals who can actually help you. Next to quitting smoking (if you have that particular habit), losing excess weight should be the most important item on your health agenda.

7

THE FIFTH KEY:
GET MOVING

Regular exercise is a cornerstone of healthy living and weight loss for a number of reasons:

- Exercise builds (or at least maintains) muscle, which utilizes more fuel in its daily operations than fat does.
- When you are burning more calories than you are eating, your body may begin mobilizing protein in muscle as fuel, rather than tapping into fat stores. Exercise builds muscle mass and in so doing helps to limit this unwanted effect.
- Exercise reduces the risk of developing coronary artery disease, cancer, and diabetes, all of which are hazards of being overweight or obese. Exercise is also crucial to controlling type 2 diabetes.
- Exercise increases alertness, energy, and general well-being, all of which can improve one's ability to resist poor food choices or eating to relieve stress or boredom. (*I just walked two miles this morning—I don't want to blow my progress by eating this doughnut.*)

As part of your weight-management program, you should set a goal to do some moderate aerobic exercise (such as walking, cycling, or swimming) for thirty min-

utes at least five days per week and do a simple
strength-training routine two or three times per week.

WHAT KIND OF EXERCISE SHOULD I BE DOING?

First steps (literally)—the basics

The first priority for the person who is exercising rarely
or not at all is to *get started on a consistent routine of aerobic activity*. (When our heart, lungs, and circulation
keep up with our body's demand for oxygen we are
said to be functioning on an aerobic—literally, "with
oxygen"—basis.) This is the simplest type of exercise to
begin and the one most likely to have an immediate
impact. Unless you have had a major injury or other
physical handicap, for example, it doesn't take any
training, experience, or special equipment to begin
walking. But how much aerobic exercise—walking or
otherwise—should you be doing? This question has
been addressed by a number of national organizations
(such as the National Institutes of Health, the American
Heart Association, and the American College of Sports
Medicine) over the past few decades, and the answer
has evolved significantly over that time. Recommendations in the 1970s and 1980s reflected the notion that
exercise had to be both frequent and strenuous in
order to benefit the heart and general health. A more
recent consensus, however, is that we can obtain significant health benefits from physical activity that is less

intense. The current wisdom may be summarized as follows:

1. **Every adult and child should attempt to accumulate thirty minutes of moderate-intensity physical activity on most, if not all, days of the week.** We may have different ideas of what constitutes moderate-intensity activity. Is it a couple of laps through the mall? mowing the lawn? running a mile? Current advisories from the National Center for Chronic Disease Prevention and Health Promotion define a moderate amount of physical activity as that which burns approximately 150 calories over the course of a day, or roughly one thousand calories per week.

2. **It is not necessary for all thirty minutes of activity to be carried out at the same time, nor do they all have to involve the same type of exercise.** The benefits of exercise can be obtained through two 15-minute, or even three 10-minute, periods of activity. Furthermore, many people prefer to vary the type of exercise they do from day to day, or even within the same day, to prevent boredom.

3. **Consistency counts.** In order to obtain—and maintain—health benefits, moderate physical activity should be on the agenda every day—or nearly every day. The weekend warrior who shuns exercise during the week and then goes "pedal to the metal"

Some Moderate-Intensity Activities

LESS VIGOROUS, MORE TIME

- Washing and waxing a car for 45–60 minutes
- Washing windows or floors for 45–60 minutes
- Playing volleyball for 45 minutes
- Playing touch football for 30–45 minutes
- Gardening for 30–45 minutes
- Wheeling self in wheelchair for 30–40 minutes
- Walking 1¾ miles in 35 minutes (20 min/mile)
- Shooting baskets for 30 minutes
- Bicycling 5 miles in 30 minutes
- Dancing fast for 30 minutes
- Pushing a stroller 1½ miles in 30 minutes
- Raking leaves for 30 minutes
- Walking 2 miles in 30 minutes (15 min/mile)
- Doing water aerobics for 30 minutes
- Swimming laps for 20 minutes
- Playing wheelchair basketball for 20 minutes
- Playing basketball for 15–20 minutes
- Bicycling 4 miles in 15 minutes
- Jumping rope for 15 minutes
- Running 1½ miles in 15 minutes (10 min/mile)
- Shoveling snow for 15 minutes
- Stair walking for 15 minutes

MORE VIGOROUS, LESS TIME

Source: Centers for Disease Control and Prevention

on Saturday, pushing heart and muscles to their limit, is likely to strain, sprain, or break something sooner or later. More importantly, he or she is *less* likely to reap the health benefits of physical activity than the person who puts forth more consistent but less vigorous effort.

Beyond entry level: pushing your envelope

Increasing the frequency, duration, and/or intensity of aerobic exercise can have a number of distinctive payoffs:

Improved overall health. The health benefits outlined at the beginning of this chapter are enhanced. In general, those who exercise harder, longer, and more often tend to live longer, have fewer heart attacks, are less prone to develop diabetes, and so on. Obviously, there is a limit to this benefit. Like anything else in life, there *can* be too much of a good thing. It isn't wise to run sixteen hours a day, for example. Also, keep in mind that *the most significant health benefits occur when we get off the couch and shift from sedentary living to consistent moderate exercise.*

Enhanced well-being. With rare exception, a dramatic improvement in overall well-being is associated with increased aerobic fitness. Energy, focus, productivity, and mood are all enhanced.

Personal satisfaction. There is a real sense of accomplishment when we see some progress, when we reach a goal, when we discover that we can do more than we thought. Ask anyone who has completed a marathon for the first time—no matter how long it took to cover the 26.2-mile course—and you will hear about a rush of emotion at the finish line that far over-shadows any sore muscles. Nevertheless, some cautions are worth noting.

Keep it safe

If you have been doing a basic moderate workout (for example, a thirty-minute walk at three to four miles per hour) consistently five days per week, keep the follow-ing in mind:

1. **Get medical clearance** if you are a man over forty or a woman over fifty, or if you have risk factors for (or symptoms remotely suggesting) heart disease.

2. **Make changes gradually in order to prevent inju-ries, fatigue, and discouragement**. If you normally walk for thirty minutes, for example, you may dis-cover some new unhappy muscles if you suddenly jump to sixty minutes. You would be better off increasing the time of your walk by three to five minutes each week. If you are regularly walking two miles in forty minutes and want to speed things up, don't expect to jog or run the entire distance. Instead, after you have warmed up, try alternating jogging and walking every two or three minutes. As

your stamina improves, you will be able to increase
the amount of time you spend jogging, your pace, or
both. The same principle applies to other aerobic
exercise, whether riding a bicycle (moving or sta-
tionary), swimming, using a stair-climber machine,
and so on. Remember that your purpose is not to
push yourself to a near-death experience. If you feel
faint, dizzy, or simply unable to press on, *slow down or
stop* until you are ready to continue (or, if necessary,
call it quits for the day). Ideally you will find a
cruising speed at which your breathing can
comfortably keep up with your body's increased
need for oxygen for longer and longer periods
of time.

3. **Don't forget to warm up and cool down.** This is
   important for anyone exercising—not merely world-
   class athletes who are about to compete for a place
   on the medal platform. In fact, it is particularly
   important if you have not been exercising consistently (or at all). If your schedule is tight or your day
   long, you may be tempted to skip the warm-up or
   cooldown, which is definitely a bad idea. Five to ten
   (or even fifteen) minutes should be spent doing your
   activity of choice at a more relaxed, comfortable
   level before shifting gears to begin more serious
   exertion. If you're going to jog or run, a brisk walk
   should start your session. If you have just mounted a

bicycle, don't begin your ride by storming up the nearest hill. Your heart needs a little time to increase its rate, and your vascular system (your arteries and veins) must divert more blood to muscles that need much more oxygen as they work harder. Those muscles, and the tendons which connect them to bones, are also more prone to tear if they are suddenly called upon to give their all. If you want to stretch before your workout, do it *after* you warm up in order to avoid damaging muscles. Similarly, after a period of vigorous exertion, you need to reverse the events that took place during your warm-up. Your heart needs to slow down gradually, and blood needs to be shunted from your muscles to other parts of the body. A sudden shift from "sixty to zero" could cause enough of a drop in blood pressure to make you dizzy or even faint. Some gentle stretching after your cooldown may help prevent cramping and muscle tightness.

4. **If you develop chest pain during any workout— even one you have previously tolerated—stop immediately.** If the pain does not go away within a few minutes, call 911 or have someone take you immediately to the nearest hospital emergency room. If the pain subsides relatively quickly, talk to your doctor before you resume your exercise pro-

gram. Not all chest pain is a distress signal from the heart, but this symptom must not be ignored.

5. **Use your pulse to guide the pace of your activity.** You no doubt know that your heart beats more rapidly during exercise, but how fast should it go? If you have a heart condition or take any medication that affects your heart's response to exercise, you will need guidance from your doctor (or possibly a cardiologist) on this topic. Otherwise, it's useful to know your target heart rate, which you can use to estimate how hard this all-important organ is working. Most experts maintain that you benefit most from exercise when your pulse stays between 50 percent and 75 percent of your maximum heart rate, which is calculated by subtracting your age from the number 220. You probably won't expend a tremendous amount of energy to reach the lower end of the target zone, and you may feel that you are putting forth Olympian effort to keep it at the upper level. Beginners should stay near the 50 percent mark for a few weeks. They may then gradually increase the intensity of exertion over the next several months until their heart rate approaches the 75 percent level for most of the workout (after an appropriate warm-up, of course). If you've been exercising consistently for six months and have been able to exercise comfortably at the 75 percent level,

you may consider pushing up to 85 percent of your maximum rate.

A FEW WAYS TO MAKE EXERCISE MORE SATISFYING (AND CONSISTENT)

A highly disciplined person may be willing to submit to a daily exercise routine that he or she truly dislikes. For the other 98 percent of us, it helps if we can make the process as enjoyable as possible. Here are some suggestions:

Exercise with another person. Walk and talk with your spouse; you may find that the opportunity to debrief on a regular basis is habit-forming. Bike, hike, or play vigorously with your kids; to you it may be just a workout, but for them every one of these experiences builds powerful bonds and memories. Set times to exercise with a friend; not only will you enjoy each other's company, but you will be less likely to skip it if you know that someone is waiting for you. When planning social events with friends, consider options beyond merely talking and eating. Try recreational sports such as tennis or golf.

Pay attention to the setting. Is your walking route pleasant and peaceful or polluted and noisy? If you buy a treadmill or a set of weights, do you have to stare at paint cans and boxes in the garage, illuminated by a bare bulb hanging from the ceiling, while you use it? If you're thinking about joining a gym, is it a place you find inviting or a moldy den of sweat strictly for the die-hard bodybuilders? You may not have unlimited options about your surroundings, but you should be able to find a pleasant setting in which to exercise. For example, if there's too much traffic whizzing by, too many unruly dogs running loose, or too many steep hills to climb in the vicinity of your home or apartment, consider driving to a park—or another neighborhood—to go walking or jogging. Many malls open their doors early in the day to offer exercisers a safe, well-lit, and temperate environment.

You don't have to be bored (part 1). Some people lose their enthusiasm when their exercise becomes more of a rut than a routine—the same walking path, the same workout video, and so on. As we saw earlier in the chapter, there are many ways to move your muscles—and that list doesn't even include strengthening and flexibility exercises. Not only can you vary the type of activity, but also the location, time of day, and companion(s): human, animal, or none at all.

You don't have to be bored (part 2). If you're on your own during a workout, the time you spend can be put to use in more ways than one. In the midst of a hectic day, your exercise time may be your one opportunity to think—to process what's going on in your life without distraction. Many people find that their prayer is more focused during exercise, especially when walking or jogging. (If you have enough breath to pray out loud, your train of thought may take even fewer detours.) Portable tape, CD, or MP3 players are now quite inexpensive, and hearing your favorite music while you exercise is a great motivator to keep moving. Better yet, a riveting audiobook can help time pass very quickly. Many public libraries have scores of books on tape or CD, or they can be rented for a modest fee from a number of companies.

Establish everyday habits that increase your activity level. Here are some ideas:

- Take the stairs instead of the elevator or escalator.
- Don't play "chicken" with other drivers for that hotly contested parking space near the entrance to the mall. Deliberately park some distance away (where there are plenty of spaces) and walk.
- If you have to run an errand that isn't too far away, walk or ride a bike.
- Get a cordless phone with a headset so that you can walk around while talking rather than sitting in one place.
- Do your own yard work—or at least some of it.
- If you travel on business, try to stay at hotels that have a fitness center or pool, and make use of these amenities.
- For physical, intellectual, emotional, and spiritual reasons, the time your kids spend staring at the television, playing video games, or using the computer for recreation should be limited to two hours per day. The same goes for you.

AN IMPORTANT REALITY CHECK

There is no question that exercise makes a vital contribution to your overall well-being and the efficiency of your weight-loss efforts. However, it is very unlikely that thirty to sixty minutes of exercise every day *by itself* will make a rapid dent in your weight. A brisk walk, for example, burns only about one hundred calories per mile. But your body fat, a terrifically efficient form of fuel storage, stores roughly 3,500 calories per pound. A little arithmetic indicates that if you decide to lose weight by walking without changing your eating habits, you need to cover thirty-five miles for every pound of fat you want to shed. If what you're eating is maintaining a stable weight and you begin walking two miles five to seven days every week, you'll lose between one and two pounds every month. Over time this adds up (so by all means keep it up), and ten to twenty pounds lost over the course of a year can offer some important benefits to your health—but it may not be as fast a rate of loss as you'd like.

8

A FINAL THOUGHT: THE BOTTOM LINE AND THE BIG PICTURE

If you flipped to the end of this book without reading what came first, hoping to find the single answer that will make your weight problem go away, you will be disappointed. If you have read this material carefully, you'll understand why someone looking for that one bottom line is taking the wrong approach.

There are many reasons why America is in the midst of an obesity epidemic. There are also two important reasons why efforts to lose weight so frequently fail:

1. We try to make it too simple. Specifically, we want a quick fix, a miracle cure, a single food (or food group) to eat or avoid that will make our fat go away, without looking carefully at how our life, our habits, our needs, even our hurts affect our eating.

2. We try to make it too complicated. We become fixated on whether or not to eat this type of fruit or that cut of meat, or whether we can combine one

type of food with another. Some families are divided at the dinner table over various members' allegiances to a particular dietary school of thought, missing opportunities for intimacy and harmony. Yes, there are clearly ways to eat smarter, but eventually the problem boils down to figuring out how to be satisfied with fewer calories and how to increase the amount of activity we engage in every day.

Achieving and maintaining a healthy weight requires a steady, livable, step-by-step, day-by-day effort. It usually involves work on multiple fronts, including food choices and quantities, exercise, environment, habits, and emotions. With rare exception it also requires more of our time than we would really like to give, which means that it may be necessary to make some fundamental changes in schedules, activities, and (above all) expectations. But the long-term benefits are definitely worth the effort. And, of equal importance, *anyone* can make these changes. A person doesn't need to be a nutritionist, a marathon runner, or a psychologist to bring them about. You do not need a will of steel, nor must you endure endless (or even short-term) hunger, to lose weight. Remember an important word in the first sentence of this paragraph: *livable*. What ultimately works are the adjustments that a person can live with indefinitely.

Index

GET THE *COMPLETE GUIDE TO FAMILY HEALTH, NUTRITION & FITNESS!*

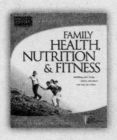

This comprehensive guide will help you take an active role in improving your health and well-being, as well as that of your entire family. It offers authoritative and current medical information in a convenient, easy-to-understand format. Taking a balanced, commonsense approach to the issue of health and wellness, this indispensable guide delivers helpful resources with an encouraging perspective.

OTHER FAITH AND FAMILY STRENGTHENERS FROM FOCUS ON THE FAMILY®

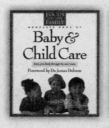

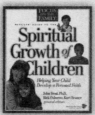

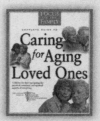

$6 REBATE

....

For a limited time you can get a $6.00 rebate on your purchase of *Complete Guide to Family Health, Nutrition, and Fitness*. Book must have been purchased in a retail store to qualify. Just return the completed rebate form, the original dated store receipt, and a photocopy of the UPC bar code from the book to: Complete Guide Rebate, Attn. Customer Service, 351 Executive Dr., Carol Stream, IL 60188.

Name: _____

Address: _____

_____

City: _____ State: _____ Zip: _____

Store where purchased: _____

E-mail address: _____

Signature: _____

DISCARD